Study Guide for
Nichols and Zwelling

MATERNAL-NEWBORN NURSING
Theory and Practice

by **THELMA PATRICK, PhD, RN**

Research Associate
Magee-Womens Research Institute
Pittsburgh, Pennsylvania

with contributions by Francine Nichols, PhD, RNC, FACCE
President, MCH Consultants, Washington, D.C.

W.B. SAUNDERS COMPANY
A Division of Harcourt Brace & Company
Philadelphia   London   Toronto   Montreal   Sydney   Tokyo

W. B. SAUNDERS COMPANY
A Division of Harcourt Brace & Company

The Curtis Center
Independence Square West
Philadelphia, PA 19106-3399

Study Guide for Nichols and Zwelling
Maternal-Newborn Nursing: Theory and Practice   ISBN 0–7216–6258–7

Printed in the United States of America

Last digit is the print number: 9   8   7   6   5   4   3   2   1

Preface

This study guide was prepared to reinforce content and enhance the understanding of the role of the nurse in maternal-newborn nursing practice as presented in the text *MATERNAL NEWBORN NURSING: THEORY AND PRACTICE* by Francine H. Nichols and Elaine Zwelling. The purpose of this study guide is to help the student focus on the most important content and to apply principles and concepts learned to patient care and nursing practice. Through the use of this study guide, the student will reinforce her or his knowledge about care of the obstetric patient and newborn and consider the more complex social, cultural, and legal issues that influence the care of the women throughout childbearing.

The study guide is primarily a tool for study, thus the exercises include short answers, multiple choice, and matching. Clinical situations, care planning techniques, and comparative analysis of realities of practice setting with the philosophies and standards of practice provide opportunities for classroom or conference dialogue.

For the instructor who has adopted the text, the study guide can be used to lead classroom discussion, prepare short oral quizzes, and to plan for pre and post clinical group sessions. Answers to questions in this study guide are printed in *Instructor's Manual for Maternal-Newborn Nursing: Theory and Practice*. Although some students working independently would prefer to have the answers in the study guide, instructors who assign exercises have asked us to print answers only in the instructor's manual. Instructors who have adopted the text for use may photocopy and distribute answers to students in their classes, in accordance with copyright guidelines printed in the instructor's manual.

Note, too, in the front of the text, a special section to inform and assist the student and instructor in learning how to use the World Wide Web to obtain information on maternal newborn nursing practices, statistics, and all the latest news from researchers.

Contents

UNIT 6: Nursing Care of Mothers and Newborns with Special Needs

Using the World Wide Web to Obtain Information

STUDY OBJECTIVES

1. Discuss how the World Wide Web can be used as an information resource for nursing practice.

2. Demonstrate how to obtain specific information from health-related web sites.

3. Compare pregnancy and parenting information from different web sites for credibility, accuracy, and appropriateness for expectant and new parents.

4. Locate resources that you could use in presenting a clinical conference on positioning during labor.

5. Explore nursing resources on the World Wide Web.

6. Subscribe to a maternal-newborn nursing mailing list.

WORKSHEET

The World Wide Web is a massive treasure chest of information. It also provides virtually instant access via mailing lists (also called listservs) to maternal-child health professionals throughout the world. Connecting to the World Wide Web has been described as "walking into an international bazaar . . . there are shops and stalls, nooks and crannies, broad avenues, back alleys, and secret passages." (Glossbrenner and Glossbrenner, 1994) For example, with the click of your mouse, you can go to the World Health Organization in Switzerland, the Centers for Disease Control in Atlanta, Georgia, or AWHONN in Washington, DC, to obtain information on the topic you are studying.

The exercises in this section are an introduction to information resources that are available on the World Wide Web. When you have completed these exercises, you will know how to access information on the web with greater efficiency. The information on the web is constantly changing, and new information is added daily. If you cannot access a web site using the Internet address that has been given, do a search for it using the name of the web site. If you need basic information on how to use the World Wide Web, consult a text on how to use the Internet.

Now, access the Internet and get ready to "surf" the web!

1. Visit the ***Association of Women's Health, Obstetric and Neonatal Nurses (AWHONN)*** home page by entering http://www.awhonn.org/ in the box for the Internet address.

    a. Describe the current nursing issues presented on the AWHONN web site.

    b. Select "Resources." Find "Practice," and select "Position Statements." What is the AWHONN position on nursing responsibilities related to intrapartum fetal heart rate monitoring?

    c. On the "Resources" page, select "FAX on Demand" and review the information that is available. Order one article that you could use to develop a teaching plan for new parents. Order one article that you could use to develop a clinical conference on maternity nursing for your peers. Share the information you found with your peers in clinical conference.

    d. What are AWHONN's current advocacy activities? How can you become involved?

2. Go to the ***Centers for Disease Control and Prevention (CDC)*** web site by entering http://www.cdc.gov/ in the Internet address box. Review the different types of information that are available from the agency.

    a. Select "MMWR." Search for information on perinatal group B streptococcal disease. How many mothers and infants are affected by this disease yearly?

b. Select "MMWR Recommendations and Reports" on the MMWR page. Find the May 31, 1996, report "Prevention of Perinatal Group B Streptococcal Disease: A public health perspective." What two approaches does this report give for the treatment of perinatal group B streptococcal disease? Do a search to determine if this is the most recent information on recommended treatment of the disease.

3. Go to the ***National Center for Health Statistics (NCHS)*** web site by entering http://www.cdc.gov/nchswww/nchshome.htm in the Internet address box. The NCHS web site can also be accessed from the CDC home page by selecting "Data and Statistics."

   a. Select the White House Social Statistics Briefing Room. On this page, select Health Statistics. List the key information included on this page.

   b. Develop a plan for improving the health status of a community using the information from the "Health Statistics."

c. Return to the first page of the NCHS web site. Select "Data Warehouse." Under "Statistical Tables," select "Published Tables." How many vaginal, cesarean, and VBAC births have there been for the last three years of published data?

4. Go to the ***World Health Organization (WHO)*** in Geneva, Switzerland, by entering http://www.who.org/ in the Internet address box.

a. Read the World Health Report. Describe the status of child mortality in the world today. What has WHO done to improve infant, child, and adolescent health? What recommendations does WHO have to improve infant, child, and adolescent health?

b. Do a search using the key word "breastfeeding." Read the WHO press release of August 6, 1996, called "World Breastfeeding Week 1996." Describe how you could use the information to develop a breastfeeding education program for maternal-newborn professionals.

5. Go to the ***OBGYN.net*** web site by entering http://www.obgyn.net in the Internet address box. Select "Forums: Discussion." Do a search by entering the key word "episiotomy."

a. Read Dr. Michael Klein's post of March 11, 1996. In his study, what did he find were a woman's chances of having severe perineal trauma if the woman had an episiotomy? If the woman did not have an episiotomy?

b. Review the other posts on episiotomy. What are your conclusions on the risks of episiotomy?

6. Compare the pregnancy and parenting information for expectant and new parents on the three web sites listed below. Evaluate the credibility of the authors and the information, the accuracy of the information, and the appropriateness of the information for parents. Give the rationale for each of your decisions.
    - *Pampers Total Baby Care*   http://pampers.com/
    - *The Whole Nine Months*   http://homearts.com/
      (Select "Family Time" then select "The Whole Nine Months")
    - *Family Internet Home Page*   http://www.familyinternet.com/ babycare/babycare.htm

Web Site	Credibility	Accuracy	Appropriateness
Pampers Total Baby Care Who wrote the articles? Would you recommend this web site to parents?	Of Author(s)? Of Content?		
The Whole Nine Months Who wrote the articles? Would you recommend this web site to parents?	Of Author(s)? Of Content?		
Family Internet Home Page Who wrote the articles? Would you recommend this web site to parents?	Of Author(s)? Of Content?		

7. Go to the ***Childbirth Resources*** web site by entering http://www.jashford.com/birth.html in the Internet address box. Develop a clinical conference on positioning during labor using resources described in this website.

8. Do a search using Alta Vista, Excite, or another search engine using the key word "nursing." Review the nursing resource web sites you located during the search. Which are your favorite sites? Which web sites give you access to a free medline search of the literature? Be sure to check out the ***MCH, The American Journal of Maternal/Child Nursing*** located at http://www.ajn.org/mcn/page1.html.

9. Subscribe to the perinatal nurses' mailing list by sending an e-mail to:
    LISTSERV@ubvm.cc.buffalo.edu
    Enter the following message in the message text area:
    subscribe pnatalrn yourfirstname yourlastname
    Leave the subject line blank.

    a. Read all of the posts for one week. List the primary topics of discussion. What have you learned from reading the posts?

    b. List three ways that being a member of this mailing list can help you in your practice.

REFERENCE

Glossbrenner, A. and Glossbrenner, E. (1994). *Internet Slick Tricks.* New York: Random House, page 6.

Chapter 1

Maternal-Newborn Nursing Science

STUDY OBJECTIVES

1. Discuss the utility of research to maternal-newborn nursing practice.

2. Identify theories that provide guidance in maternal-newborn nursing practice.

3. Define *basic research* and *applied research*.

4. Differentiate basic research from applied research.

5. Identify the steps in the research process.

6. Identify three organizations that establish research priorities for maternal-newborn nursing research.

WORKSHEET

1. In general, theory provides useful guidance for nursing practice. List five ways in which theory is useful to the maternal-newborn nurse.

2. Match the following clinical observations (Column A) with the theory that may provide guidance for practice (Column B)

<table>
<tr><th>Column A
Clinical Observation or Problem</th><th>Column B
Theory that May Assist the Nurse</th></tr>
<tr><td>1. ____ A new mother confides that she is very insecure about caring for her infant at home. She inquires about support groups or community agencies that she can call if she has concerns.</td><td>A. Nichols noted that adolescents respond differently than adult women to childbirth; he developed a model to describe the adolescent childbirth experience.</td></tr>
<tr><td>2. ____ The nurse identifies concerns for infant welfare and seeks a method of assessing the environmental and physiological risk to the infant in hopes of prescribing preventive action.</td><td>B. A "sensitive period" for the development of mother and infant attachment was described by Klaus and Kennell.</td></tr>
<tr><td>3. ____ Judy would like to know more about how the age of a mother influences her parenting experience.</td><td>C. Rubin's theory on maternal role attainment emphasizes the psychological operations involved in achieving maternal identity.

D. Mercer identified a number of key variables that may influence a woman's successful attainment of the maternal role.</td></tr>
<tr><td>4. ____ A mother inquires about the importance of frequent contact with her infant in the first several days of life.</td><td>E. Barnard's Child Health Assessment Model assesses perinatal, parental, child characteristics and parent-child interaction factors that shape child development.</td></tr>
<tr><td>5. ____ A nurse has been asked to assess the need for a special childbirth preparation class for pregnant adolescents.</td><td></td></tr>
</table>

3. Define the following terms:

Basic research:

Applied research:

4. From the following list, identify the research that is Basic (**B**) and Applied (**A**) by placing the correct letter in the blank preceding the description of research.

_____ Family stresses preceding preterm birth

_____ Spouses' pregnancy related experiences

_____ Extrauterine stimulation for preterm infants

_____ The effect of discharge time on cost and quality of care for high-risk infants

_____ Maternal role attainment

_____ Positions for childbirth

_____ Smoking cessation during pregnancy

_____ Maternal self-care

5. Identify the three organizations that establish research priorities for maternal-newborn nursing research.

6. Identify a clinical problem from maternal-newborn nursing that you would like to study. List the steps you would take to develop and implement a research study for this problem.

Chapter 2

Perspectives on Maternal-Newborn Nursing

STUDY OBJECTIVES

1. Define *maternal-newborn nursing*.

2. Define rates that serve as indicators of maternal-infant health.

3. Identify women at risk for negative maternal-newborn outcomes.

4. Identify primary, secondary, and tertiary levels of care.

5. Discuss the need for standards of care in nursing practice.

6. Identify organizations that establish standards for maternal-newborn practice.

7. Discuss the purpose of a collaborative care map.

8. Identify sources of health care goals for maternal-newborn health.

9. Identify actions that can be taken by the individual to improve maternal-newborn health.

10. Discuss criteria for the decision regarding hospital versus home birth.

WORKSHEET

1. Define *maternal-newborn nursing*.

2. Match each term in Column A with the appropriate definition in Column B.

Column A	**Column B**

Column A

____ Birth rate

____ Live birth

____ Maternal mortality rate

____ Neonatal mortality rate

____ Low birthweight

____ Preterm birth

____ Infant mortality rate

Column B

A. Birth after fewer than 37 completed weeks gestation

B. The number of deaths of infants under one year of age per 1,000 live births

C. The number of births per 1,000 population

D. Weight of less than 2,500 grams at birth

E. An infant who after birth demonstrates evidence of life, including heartbeat, pulsation of the umbilical cord, and movement of voluntary muscles

F. The number of deaths for infants under 28 days per 1,000 live births

G. The number of deaths of women from complications of pregnancy, childbirth, and the postpartum period per 100,000 live births

3. Using the letters in front of these age- and racially defined groups, identify those groups for whom these rates are likely to be higher. (There may be more than one response per maternal-infant health indicator.)

A. Women over 30

B. Adolescents

C. Black women

D. Hispanic women

E. White women

____ Infant mortality

____ Neonatal mortality

____ Low birthweight

____ Maternal mortality

____ Birth rate

4. Which of the following is an example of *primary* care?
   A. A smoking cessation program for pregnant women
   B. A preconception health class
   C. Counseling a teenager who is pregnant
   D. Providing nursing care to a woman with preeclampsia

5. Which of the following is an example of *secondary* care?
   A. A smoking cessation program for pregnant women
   B. A preconception health class
   C. Counseling a teenager who is pregnant
   D. Providing nursing care to a woman with preeclampsia

6. What is a nursing standard?

7. What purpose do nursing standards have in nursing practice?

8. Name two organizations that have developed standards for maternal-newborn nursing.

9. What is certification? Is certification different from licensure? Explain.

10. List two purposes of a collaborative care map.

11. What is *Healthy People 2000?*

12. List three of the measures recommended to reduce infant mortality, and indicate an action you, as an individual, can take to contribute to improved outcomes.

Measures	Action
1.	1.
2.	2.
3.	3.

13. Discuss Table 2-3, Infant Mortality Rates for Industrialized Countries. What factors might contribute to the United States' standing on that chart?

14. Identify three beliefs that are central to maternal-newborn nursing practice.

15. Jessica, a close friend, calls you to announce that she is pregnant. She is trying to decide if she should seek care for her pregnancy and delivery within an obstetric practice with a hospital delivery or with a midwife with the possibility of a home birth.

    Considering that Jessica is of good health, what criteria would you provide to Jessica so that she can assess these two possibilities?

16. List three advantages and three disadvantages of single-room maternity care (SRMC).

Chapter 3

Roles of the Maternal-Newborn Nurse

STUDY OBJECTIVES

1. Identify changes in the health care system that influence the role of the maternal-newborn nurse.

2. Identify role dimensions that may be a part of the professional nurse's role.

3. Differentiate core and functional role dimensions.

4. Identify ways in which the nurse and the case manager can collaborate to accomplish efficient and effective nursing care.

5. Discuss experiences, education, and role expectations for selected advanced practice roles.

WORKSHEET

1. Stolte and colleagues (1994) assessed maternal-newborn nurses' perceptions about changes in maternity care. For each of these eight observed changes, listed in order of frequency of report, consider the implications for the care you provide.

   a. Increased use of technology

   b. Increased emphasis on the legal aspects of care

   c. Shorter patient stays

   d. Increased emphasis on cost containment

   e. Increased involvement of the family in the birth process

f. Cross training so that the nurse can function in multiple maternal-newborn areas

g. Increased consumer demand for childbirth education and childbirth options

h. Implementation of single-room maternity care

2. Identify each role dimension as a core or functional dimension by placing a **C** (for *core*) or an **F** (for *functional*) on the line provided.

____ Advocate		____ Change agent	
____ Expertise		____ Critical thinking	
____ Educator		____ Political activist	
____ Manager		____ Problem solver	
____ Caregiver		____ Researcher	

3. Within your community, locate a certified nurse midwife, a certified nurse practitioner, or a clinical nurse specialist who practices in maternal-newborn nursing. Ask for an opportunity to discuss how that professional chose and became prepared for that role, what the professional perceives to be the primary functions of that role, and what advice that professional would have for a nurse considering a future in that role. Summarize your discussion in the space below.

4. It is projected that the role of case manager will be a career opportunity for nurses in this area of managed care. A case manager is responsible for decreasing costs by eliminating unnecessary services, while ensuring that patients receive appropriate and timely care. List any observations you have made regarding situations or areas in maternal-newborn care in which you judge these goals can be addressed.

5. Ask for an opportunity to discuss case management in maternal-newborn care with a person who is a case manager. Identify three aspects of maternal-newborn care that are of special interest to the case manager to accomplish efficient, effective care in maternal-newborn settings.

Chapter 4

Family Dynamics

STUDY OBJECTIVES

1. Identify various family formations.

2. Discuss changes in family units in relation to birth, marriage, definition of family, and roles of family members.

3. List the major functions of the family.

4. Identify characteristics of blended families.

5. Identify activities that may help the blended family attain integration.

6. List developmental tasks for the adoptive family.

7. Compare the educational needs of childbearing and adoptive families.

8. Identify and describe various family theories.

9. Identify and describe the factors that influence family functioning.

10. Describe the theoretical foundations of two family assessment tools.

11. Discuss reliability and validity of instrumentation in research.

12. Describe responsibilities outlined in the blueprint for national family policy as specified by the National Commission on Children.

WORKSHEET

1. Match the family form in Column A with the appropriate definition in Column B.

<table>
<tr><td align="center">**Column A**</td><td>**Column B**</td></tr>
<tr><td>1. _____ Extended family</td><td>A. Husband and wife or other couple living alone without children</td></tr>
<tr><td>2. _____ Dyad</td><td></td></tr>
<tr><td>3. _____ Nuclear family</td><td>B. One or both spouses have been divorced or widowed and have married into a family with at least one child</td></tr>
<tr><td>4. _____ Step-parent</td><td></td></tr>
<tr><td>5. _____ Cohabiting</td><td>C. A homosexual couple living together with or without children; children may be adopted, from previous relationships, or artificially conceived</td></tr>
<tr><td>6. _____ Gay</td><td></td></tr>
<tr><td>7. _____ No-kin</td><td></td></tr>
<tr><td></td><td>D. Three generations, including married brothers and sisters and their families</td></tr>
<tr><td></td><td>E. A father, mother, and child living together but apart from both sets of their parents</td></tr>
<tr><td></td><td>F. An unmarried couple living together</td></tr>
<tr><td></td><td>G. A group of at least two people sharing a relationship and exchanging support who have no legalized or blood ties to each other</td></tr>
</table>

2. Discuss changes in the American family in relation to the following items.

    a. Birth

    b. Marriage

    c. Definition and structure of family

    d. Role of the mother

    e. Roles of children

    f. Role of the father

3. Name five major functions of the family.

   a.

   b.

   c.

   d.

   e.

4. Please complete the following statements regarding characteristics of successful blended families.

   a. Individual family members _____ attempt to force their blended family into the mold of a traditional nuclear family.
   b. Children are likely to exhibit their grief with their blended family status through behaviors such as _____, _____, and
   _____.
   c. According to Reutter and Strang (1986), integration of stepfamilies may take as long as _____ years.
   d. The three major issues of concern to blended families are _____
   _____, _____,
   and _____.

5. Identify three activities that you might suggest to a blended family to help family members achieve the goal of successful integration.

6. List six critical developmental tasks for an adoptive family.

7. How do the educational needs of the childbearing family and the adoptive family compare? Name three specific classes that you would want to present for an adoptive family.

8. Identify the statement that describes each theory by placing the appropriate letter on the line before each statement.

____ As transitions occur within the family, a growth responsibility arises in the life of the family. Failure to achieve certain growth responsibilities will be apparent in later family life.

A. Symbolic Interaction Theory

B. Family Developmental Theory

C. Family Systems Theory

D. Social Exchange Theory

____ Individuals are perceived as making choices to result in the greatest reward and least cost regarding material and non-material concerns, as in status and relationships.

____ The family is an emotional relationship system made up of interlocking systems and subsystems.

____ The internal process of assigning meaning to symbols or gestures is important in determining and understanding behaviors of individuals and families. An individual's behavior is a result of the individual's perception of experiences with society.

9. Describe how the following factors influence family functioning:

    a. Power

    b. Interaction patterns

    c. Culture

    d. Values

10. Family assessment tools provide a framework for the nurse to gather information about the family that will be useful in planning care. Two commonly used assessment tools are the _____ and the _____. Complete the following table about the nature of information or outcome that is addressed by each of these instruments.

Assessment or Outcome	Family Assessment Tool
Identifies family adaptability as structured, flexible, chaotic, or rigid.	
Assesses five areas of family function: adaptation, partnership, growth, affection, and resolve.	
Identifies the individual's perception of the family's level of function.	
Derived from a family systems model.	

11. When considering using a family assessment tool such as the Family Apgar, one must be concerned about the reliability and validity of the instrument.

   a. Define *reliability*.

   b. Define *validity*.

   c. What are the common tests done and values reported to indicate an appropriate level of reliability?

12. The National Commission on Children was created by Congress and the President in 1987. In 1991, the Commission approved a comprehensive blueprint for a national family policy. In that policy, several people and groups are identified as having responsibility for meeting the needs of children. Identify the responsibilities of each of the following entities.

   a. Parents

   b. Family

   c. Community institutions

   d. Communities

   e. Society

Chapter 5

Maternal-Newborn Nursing in the Community

STUDY OBJECTIVES

1. Discuss the purpose of a home visit for the maternal-newborn nurse.

2. Identify functional role dimensions that are central to community nursing.

3. Identify the purpose of a family assessment as part of a home or community visit.

4. Organize the activities involved in preparing for and conducting a home visit.

5. Identify strategies for risk management in the practice of community nursing.

6. Identify the scope of various aspects of community assessment, and give potential sources of information for each.

7. For a sample case, identify nursing actions and necessary communications to the primary health care provider.

8. Identify concerns for practicing maternal-newborn nursing within the community, and develop a plan for resolving these concerns.

WORKSHEET

1. List five purposes for home visits in maternal-newborn nursing.

2. What functional roles (see Chapter 3) are likely to be emphasized with maternal-newborn clients in community nursing?

3. List two primary reasons for conducting a family assesssment as a part of a home or community visit.

4. Place the following phases of a home visit in order of occurrence.

_____   Controlling distractions

_____   Contracting

_____   Planning for the visit

_____   Communicating with the primary health care provider

_____   Socializing

_____   Restating the contracted goals

_____   Establishing the next appointment

_____   Clarifying responsibilities for accomplishing goals

_____   Documenting the visit

5. List the four steps in risk management for maternal-newborn nursing in the community.

a.

b.

c.

d.

6. Community assessment is an important factor in community maternal-newborn nursing practice. Complete the following table, indicating the type of information that should be assessed and potential sources of that information.

Community Characteristic	Type of Information Needed	Potential Source of Information
Age distribution		
Culture		
Environment		
Housing		
Safety		
Transportation		

7. Ms. Jones is a 22-year-old single parent that you have been asked to visit in the first week postpartum. At your visit on the fifth postpartal day, Ms. Jones is cordial and responds to questions promptly and appropriately, but admits to being quite tired. She has elected to breastfeed her infant. Her mother, Mrs. Jones, is present in the home and she wants to stay with Ms. Jones to assist her. Mrs. Jones, however, states that she could be more helpful if Ms. Jones would give up the idea of breastfeeding the baby and allow Mrs. Jones to take over some of the nighttime feedings that the new infant requires. As you talk with Ms. Jones privately, you learn that Ms. Jones wants to breastfeed her infant for as long as she possibly can. In her fatigue and with uncertainties that the baby is being adequately nourished, Ms. Jones is concerned that she will not be able to assert her desire to continue breastfeeding her infant. From this information, propose nursing actions that you will implement while in this home, and prepare a communication to the primary health care provider, using the sample steps proposed in Chapter 5 (page 100) of the text.

8. There are many reasons for making visits in the homes of maternal-newborn clients. Yet nurses who consider roles within the community express concerns about practicing in the community and within the homes of clients. Some of these concerns and anxieties are listed in Chapter 5, and you may have some additional concerns. Consider your feelings regarding maternal-newborn nursing in the community, and identify the factors that concern you most. List those factors in the table below, along with an action that you might take to address each concern. For additional support in problem solving, discuss this list with your colleagues, with your faculty, or with nurses who practice within the community.

Concern Regarding Community Nursing	Action(s) to Address this Concern

Chapter 6

Social Issues and Childbearing Women

STUDY OBJECTIVES

1. Define the "feminization of poverty."

2. Identify ways in which a nurse can be politically active.

3. Identify stressors experienced by clients in impoverished communities.

4. Identify relationships between prenatal care and pregnancy outcomes.

5. List physical and emotional symptoms of spouse abuse.

6. Identify substance-specific findings regarding substance use during pregnancy.

7. Define health in a manner consistent with the *Healthy People 2000* report, and identify pregnancy-specific goals.

8. Discuss factors related to access to and provision of prenatal care services.

9. Identify behaviors likely to be observed following a rape experience.

10. Plan for the care of a client following a rape experience.

11. Identify concepts from role theory that pertain to working mothers.

12. List and describe potential negative reproductive outcomes from workplace exposure to toxic substances.

WORKSHEET

1. What is the "feminization of poverty"?

2. List several ways in which the nurse can accomplish political activism on behalf of the maternal-newborn clients.

3. Stressors experienced by those who live in poverty include:

4. Identify the direction, positive or negative, of the relationship of prenatal care to the stated outcomes.

   Comprehensive prenatal care is _____ correlated with positive pregnancy outcomes and _____ correlated with negative outcomes, such as low birthweight and infant mortality.

5. Abused women may report a variety of physical and emotional symptoms similar to those fitting the profile of post-traumatic stress disorder. Complete the following table of physical and emotional symptoms.

Physical Symptoms	Emotional Symptoms

6. During a visit to a prenatal clinic, ask the clinic staff to report the percentage of appointments made that are not attended by the client. Observe the activities within the clinic, and identify five factors that you assess may contribute to nonattendance.

   a.

   b.

c.

d.

e.

7. During a client interview, ask for the client's perception of clinic care. What features did the client identify as supportive?

   a. What features increased the likelihood that the client may not attend?

   b. How did these features compare with those non-financial barriers listed in Table 6-1.

   c. What features increased the likelihood of attendance?

   d. How did these features compare with strategies to overcome non-financial barriers listed in Table 6-2.

8. Identify the following statements as true or false.

   _____ Women who are involved in substance use are more likely to seek prenatal care.

   _____ One in four babies born each year has been exposed to harmful or illegal drugs.

   _____ Low birthweight and preterm birth are the most serious known consequences of maternal illicit drug use.

   _____ White women have a lower rate of alcohol use than African-American women.

   _____ Compared to white women, African-American women have a lower rate of cocaine use.

   _____ In 1994, NIDA reported that, in general, the rate of drug use declined during pregnancy.

   _____ Thirty-two percent of women who reported the use of one drug also used alcohol and smoked cigarettes.

9. Alcohol consumption in pregnancy is associated with increased risk for fetal alcohol syndrome. The effects of this syndrome are:

   a.

   b.

c.

d.

10. What is a safe level of consumption of alcohol during pregnancy?

11. List four negative perinatal outcomes associated with the use of cocaine.

    a.

    b.

    c.

    d.

12. List behaviors likely to be observed during each of the three phases of the rape experience.

    a. Acute phase

    b. Outward phase

    c. Reorganization phase

13. Write a nursing diagnosis and identify a goal for the client for each of the three phases of the rape experience.

    a. Acute phase

    b. Outward phase

    c. Reorganization phase

14. Write the letter of the concept from role theory that applies in each of the following scenarios.

    A. Role overload   C. Role ambiguity
    B. Role conflict   D. Role incongruity

    _____ Rachel must be at the child care center by 5 PM to pick up her infant, but her boss needs her to stay until 6 PM to assist in the details of a very important appointment.

    _____ Sally has decided that the only way she can meet the demands of her work and home responsibilities is to begin her day at 4 AM.

    _____ Joan believes that she should be at home more, and she longs for time at home with her children. However, Joan's new status as a single parent has forced her to work an increased number of hours to meet financial needs.

_____ John and Kathy are both struggling to maintain an orderly home and provide care for their infant twins. They are so busy, in fact, that they have had little time to discuss who is responsible for what. As a result, some tasks are duplicated, while others are neglected.

15. List and briefly describe five negative reproductive outcomes from workplace exposure to toxic substances:

    a.

    b.

    c.

    d.

    e.

Chapter 7

Legal Aspects of Maternal-Newborn Nursing

STUDY OBJECTIVES

1. Name the four elements that comprise a negligent act.

2. Identify situations that represent negligent care or action on the part of the nurse.

3. Discuss the doctrines of Captain of the Ship, Charitable Immunity, and Respondeat Superior.

4. Discuss negligence/malpractice insurance.

5. Define *intention*.

6. Identify five sources of standards of care.

7. Discuss responsibilities of health care providers in relation to informed consent.

8. List the legal requirements of informed consent.

9. Identify measures for risk management.

10. Identify the role of the nurse in situations in which risk is evident.

WORKSHEET

1. Four elements must be present for a court to award compensation for a charge of negligence. These four elements are:

   a.

   b.

   c.

   d.

2. Specific instances in which a nurse might be found negligent in a maternal-child setting include (circle all that apply):

   Accepting responsibility for administering Pitocin for augmentation or induction of labor without specific training about the drug.

   Turning away from an infant on an examination table.

   Failure to assess an intravenous injection site on a newborn at appropriate intervals.

   Failure to monitor the temperature of an infant in the first 24 hours, resulting in cold stress and an admission to NICU.

   The failure of a parent to place an infant in the car seat correctly, in spite of documented patient teaching and assessed comprehension of instruction.

3. Discuss the following doctrines.

   a. Captain of the Ship

   b. Charitable Immunity

   c. Respondeat Superior

4. Identify and describe the two types of negligence/malpractice insurance.

   a.

   b.

5. True or false: A nurse can obtain insurance that will protect the nurse from action or inaction that intentionally, rather than carelessly, causes harm to a person.

6. In the "eyes of the law," what is *intention* ?

7. List at least five sources of standards of care for nurses in obstetrical and newborn care.

   a.

   b.

   c.

   d.

   e.

8. Informed consent is the responsibility of the _____.

9. Legal requirements of informed consent are:

   a.

   b.

   c.

   d.

10. What is the nurse's role in relation to informed consent?

11. Measures to achieve the goal of risk management include:

   a.

   b.

   c.

   d.

12. What is the goal of risk management?

13. Mary Jo has made a medication error. She notifies the physician of the error. He judges the error to be insignificant and sees no potential harm to the patient as a result of the error. Mary Jo indicates to the physician that she will complete an incident report and leave it for the physician to review and sign. The physician tells Mary Jo that this is not necessary and tells her to "forget about it." What should Mary Jo do?

14. John, a friend, has a relative who is in your hospital. John asks that you look up his relative's diagnosis and pathology report. He is eager to know that his relative is all right.

    What legal and ethical concept would be breached in doing what John asks?

    What is an appropriate response to John?

Chapter 8

Ethical Issues in Maternal-Newborn Nursing

STUDY OBJECTIVES

1. Define *values, value systems, ethics,* and *morals*.

2. Identify ethical principles that guide decision making in nursing situations.

3. Identify the specific goals of various documents written to explicate ethical behavior.

4. Discuss the significance of the nurse's personal values to the care given to clients.

5. Differentiate ethical decision making from clinical judgment.

6. Describe methods for gaining or enhancing self-awareness.

7. Utilize a framework to gain understanding of ethical decision making in nursing practice and patient care.

WORKSHEET

1. Define the following terms.

   Values:

   Value systems:

   Ethics:

   Morals:

2. Identify the ethical principle that guides the decision or action taken by the nurse in each of these situations.

   A. Beneficence
   B. Fidelity
   C. Universality
   D. Utility

   E. Finality
   F. Confidentiality
   G. Nonmaleficence
   H. Gratitude
   I. Veracity

_____ John promised Ms. Smith that he would provide a baby-bath demonstration for her before he went home. John remained at work after his scheduled time to keep his promise.

_____ Mary assesses the injection site carefully before giving a Vitamin K injection to Baby Boy Day.

_____ Susan confides in Mary that she is considering relinquishing her infant for adoption, and thinks she would prefer to arrange an adoption through private placement. Mary has a close friend who is infertile and eager to adopt an infant. Mary does not tell her friend about the potential availability of an infant for adoption.

_____ Nancy assists Cindy with her assignment today to repay Cindy for her assistance to Nancy on a day when Nancy had a difficult assignment.

_____ Judy believes that all mothers should spend as much time as possible with their infants throughout their hospital stay. Judy organizes care so that the infant is with the mother. Judy does this for all the women she provides care to regardless of their personal circumstances, health status, or desire to be with the infant.

_____ Aware that the NICU needs additional, specialized equipment to meet infant care needs, Karen organizes a working group to identify potential financial sources for that equipment.

_____ In spite of the urgency in preparing Gloria for her cesarean section, Linda carefully repeated her instructions regarding the surgery to make certain Gloria understood the surgery and voluntarily agreed.

_____ Julia's infant is in need of a blood transfusion; however, Julia has refused this transfusion on behalf of her infant due to her own religious beliefs. In cooperation with the social worker and physician, Andrea, for the welfare of the child, petitions the court for permission to override the mother's refusal.

_____ Amy is questioned about an incident that occurred on the nursing unit. Even though she knows that her response will not reflect well on her colleagues, Amy knows she must tell the truth.

3. Match the document listed in Column A with the goal of the document in Column B.

Column A

____ American Hospital Association Patient's Bill of Rights

____ The International Childbirth Education Association Pregnant Patient's Bill of Rights

Column B

A. Identifies ethical commitment to informed, safe, competent, confidential, and considerate care for all patients

B. Ensures the pregnant patient of the right to all information about decisions that affect her health, the health of the unborn, or both

4. Discuss how a nurse's personal values might affect care given to clients.

5. Identify three documents that identify ethical *nursing* behavior.

a.

b.

c.

6. How are ethical decision making and clinical judgment different?

How are they similar?

7. Self-awareness is central to a helping relationship with a client. Describe how each of the following can assist in developing self-awareness.

a. Values clarification

b. Peer discussion

c. Life experience

d. Professional experience

e. Continuing education

On page 158 of the textbook, a model for ethical decision making is presented (see Figure 8-1). The following questions relate to that model. Circle the letter of the correct answer to each question.

8. By proximity to the nurse, what nurse and health care system factors most influence the nurse?
   a. Health care agency policies
   b. Federal policies
   c. Code of ethics
   d. The patient's prescribed medical treatment

9. Which of the following factors do sociocultural values and health care values influence?
   a. Patient and family factors
   b. Nursing and health care factors
   c. Neither patient and family nor nursing and health care factors
   d. Both patient and family and nursing and health care factors

10. Ethical dilemmas exist when there are conflicting values, obligations, or principles about the right course of action. The following are examples of situations in which nurses may find they are in conflict with the patient's values, professional values, or health care values. For each situation, identify a course of action that the nurse can take to resolve the ethical dilemma. The Perinatal-Bioethical Model for Ethical Decision Making (Figure 8-2) should provide a framework for this response.

    a. Sally, who is 15, confides to you that she is pregnant. She wishes to terminate the pregnancy, a course of action that you know is not consistent with her parents' religious beliefs, or with your own. Sally told you that it is important that her parents not know about her pregnancy, and that she is turning to you because you are a nurse and would know where she could get assistance. State law within your state would not permit Sally to have the abortion without her parents' consent, but Sally resides only 35 miles from a state in which the procedure can be done without parental consent. How would you respond to Sally?

    b. Jennifer has just been told that she is carrying a fetus that has multiple anomalies and will not likely survive following delivery. Jennifer has been advised to abort the fetus, but wonders if she can allow her pregnancy to advance to delivery, and have the chance to hold her baby. She understands that the baby has no chance for survival, and she does not want any life support measures to be implemented. The physician has not encouraged this decision, and has advised there is not precedent at the hospital for withholding intervention. Jennifer asks you for advice about who she should contact to arrange for her chosen course of action.

Chapter 9

The Reproductive System

STUDY OBJECTIVES

1. Identify the critical time for development of the reproductive system.
2. Name the purpose of the pelvis during pregnancy.
3. Identify the four pelvic types.
4. Define selected terms related to the development and structure of the reproductive system.

WORKSHEET

1. The critical period for the development of morphologic characteristics of the male and female conceptus begins at _____ weeks of gestational age.

2. List the three purposes of the pelvis during pregnancy.

   a.

   b.

   c.

3. Complete the following paragraph about pelvic types.

   There are three planes in the true pelvis: the _____, the _____, and the _____. The shape and size of these planes influence the process of labor and birth. The _____ pelvis is most favorable for successful labor and birth. Characteristics of the three planes in this pelvic type are _____.

Slow descent and midpelvic arrest can be caused by the narrow pelvic planes of the _____ pelvis. When a pelvis is determined to be _____, only the transverse diameter is adequate for passage of the fetus. The shape of the _____ _____ pelvis, seen in 25% of women, provides planes that are of adequate size for delivery.

4. Provide the correct term for each of the following definitions.

   a. The result of the XY chromosome pair _____

   b. Innervates the clitoris, the vestibule, most of the labia, and the perineum

      _____

   c. The pH of vaginal secretions _____

   d. The phase of the menstrual cycle when spiral arteries grow

      _____

   e. The phase of the menstrual cycle when spiral arteries are restricted

      _____

   f. The usual position of the uterus_____

   g. The ruptured follicle, or yellow body, that degenerates if fertilization does not occur_____

   h. Male cells that produce testosterone_____

   i. The first menstrual period _____

   j. Permanent cessation of menses _____

   k. A sex maturity rating (SMR) classification often used in assessing adolescent development_____

   l. The result of the XX chromosome pair_____

   m. Bordered by the sacrum, the innominate bones, and the pubis, this structure is the bony passage through which the fetus must pass.

      _____

   n. Tissues posterior to the labia and anterior to the anus _____

      _____

   o. Major perineal muscles of obstetric significance _____,
      _____, and_____.

   p. Cytology reading of cells from the cervix _____.

   q. Releases the follicle-stimulating and luteinizing hormones

      _____

Chapter 10

Sexuality During Pregnancy

STUDY OBJECTIVES

1. Identify components of sexual development from the fetal period through adulthood.

2. List the five primary factors in the development of adolescent sexuality.

3. Describe physical and emotional adaptations in sexual responsiveness throughout the childbearing cycle.

4. Identify the primary theories regarding sexual response and sexuality.

5. Identify measures that assist the nurse in interacting with women and men regarding sexual concerns.

WORKSHEET

1. In each blank, write the letter of the developmental stage that most closely corresponds to the developmental landmark or task.

Developmental Landmark or Task

_____ A period of rapid physical changes and stressful psychosocial demands in which achieving independence and learning social and personal responsibility are paramount.

_____ Sexual differentiation takes place, physical differences are evident.

_____ Interest is focused on elimination. Explores genitals as a part of learning about all parts of the body.

_____ Physical sexual responses are present, however, parental behaviors play a significant role in gender identity.

_____ From this time forward, learning is a stronger influence on sexual development than biology.

_____ Demonstrates pride in their learned gender identity.

_____ A time of increasing commitment and intimacy. Physical responsiveness varies with age.

_____ A feeling of omnipotence may overshadow cognitive understanding of the risks of sexual activity, such as pregnancy, sexually transmitted disease, and AIDS.

_____ In this time of increasing self-consciousness and self-awareness, it is likely that first learning about sexual intercourse will be shocking.

Developmental Stage

A. Embryonic period

B. Infancy

C. Toddler

D. Preschool

E. School-age

F. Adolescence

G. Adulthood

2. List the five primary factors in the development of adolescent sexuality.
   a.

   b.

   c.

   d.

   e.

3. Complete the following table, describing alterations in physical and emotional responsiveness throughout the childbearing cycle.

	Physical Adaptation	Psychosocial Adaptation
First Trimester		
Second Trimester		
Third Trimester		
Delivery		
Postpartum		

4. Name the researchers who have provided understanding of sexual responsiveness, and briefly describe their theories or contributions to our understanding of sexuality and sexual responsiveness.

Researcher(s)	Theory or Observation
a.	
b.	
c.	

5. List behaviors or actions that you can take to prepare for interacting with women and men about sexual responsiveness and concerns.

Chapter 11

Family Planning

STUDY OBJECTIVES

1. Define *family planning*.

2. Discuss the health, emotional, and financial benefits of family planning and the consequences of unplanned pregnancy.

3. List criteria for selecting an ideal contraceptive method.

4. Define the terms *theoretical effectiveness* and *use effectiveness*.

5. Identify the general methods of family planning as well as specific mechanisms of those methods.

6. Using criteria for selecting an ideal contraceptive method, discuss the advantages and disadvantages of various family planning methods.

7. Discuss preparation and skills maintenance for the nurse with a role in family planning.

8. Identify a nursing diagnosis and goal statement for specific situations that may be encountered when nursing practice involves family planning.

WORKSHEET

1. Define *family planning*.

2. Family planning enables physical, emotional, and financial readiness for the roles and tasks of parenthood. Discuss the potential risks of an unplanned pregnancy on the following.

   a. Health

   b. Finances

c. Psychosocial

d. Career

3. List seven criteria for the ideal contraceptive method.

a. _____

b. _____

c. _____

d. _____

e. _____

f. _____

g. _____

4. Discuss the difference between *theoretical effectiveness* and *use effectiveness*.

5. For each of the following family planning methods, indicate the mechanism and the advantages and disadvantages of that method. Consider the criteria for an ideal method in your list of advantages and disadvantages.

Method	Mechanism	Advantages	Disadvantages
Natural Family Planning			
Spermicidals			
Barrier Methods			
Intrauterine Devices			
Hormonal Contraception			

6. Assessment and teaching are primary roles of the nurse in relation to family planning. Discuss measures that the nurse should pursue to maintain competence in history taking, physical examination, and teaching.

7. Identify a nursing diagnosis and goal that might apply for women in the following "family planning" care situations.

   a. A 14-year-old teenager who is sexually active and has not been using contraception.

   b. A young adult who wishes to delay childbearing for at least 5 years.

   c. A pre-menopausal middle-aged woman who does not want to conceive again.

   d. A woman who indicates that she is having difficulty in pursuing a contraceptive because this practice conflicts with the guidance of her religious beliefs.

Chapter 12

Infertility

STUDY OBJECTIVES

1. Define *infertility*.

2. Identify factors that increase the likelihood or occurrence of infertility.

3. Identify conditions that contribute to infertility in the female and in the male.

4. Describe testing to diagnose infertility.

5. Describe usual psychosocial responses to infertility and diagnostic procedures.

WORKSHEET

1. Define *infertility*.

2. Forty percent of infertility can be expected to be due to female factors. For women, the most significant contributor to the recent increase in infertility

   is _____ . The second most frequent

   contributing factor is the physiologic consequence of _____

   _____ .

3. Male factors represent 40 percent of the occurrence of infertility. The common causes of male infertility are less well understood because multiple factors can influence the normal sperm count, motility, and morphology. List five lifestyle factors and five conditions that contribute to male infertility.

Lifestyle Factors	Other Conditions
a.	a.
b.	b.
c.	c.
d.	d.
e.	e.

4. Following a detailed history, infertility evaluation occurs in six areas. Identify the tests by the letter that apply in each of these areas. (Letters will apply to more than one phase)

_____ Ovulation

_____ Male factors

_____ Sperm-mucus interactions

_____ Tubal and uterus anatomy

_____ Endometrial insufficiency

_____ Pelvic factors

A. Basal body temperature

B. Postcoital test

C. Hysterosalpingography

D. Endometrial biopsy

E. Laparoscopy

F. Semen analysis

G. Antisperm antibodies

H. Sperm penetration test

5. Couples provide behavioral cues to their responses to aspects of diagnosis and treatment as they interact with the nurse. List several of these cues and the response that might be indicated by the cue. Suggest a statement that will allow for further assessment of the perceived response.

Cue _____

Response to therapy indicated by cue _____

Probing statement _____

_____

Cue _____

Response to therapy indicated by cue _____

Probing statement _____

_____

Cue _____

Response to therapy indicated by cue _____

Probing statement _____

_____

Cue _____

Response to therapy indicated by cue _____

Probing statement _____

_____

Chapter 13

Genetics

STUDY OBJECTIVES

1. Describe genes and chromosomes.

2. Identify tissue commonly used for genetic diagnosis.

3. Describe the occurrence of genetic mutations.

4. Define the terms *mitosis* and *meiosis*.

5. Discuss the process of gene mapping.

6. Identify common chromosomal disorders and the mechanisms that contribute to their occurrence.

7. Identify the major steps in the process of genetic counseling.

8. Identify the skills a nurse should possess if involved in genetic screening or counseling.

WORKSHEET

1. Define the following terms:

Genes

Chromosomes

Codon

Mitosis

Meiosis

2. What tissues are commonly used to determine the chromosomal constitution of an individual?

   a.

   b.

   c.

3. Discuss the importance of gene mapping in prenatal diagnosis, in carrier detection, and in exploring adult-onset disorders with a genetic component.

4. What are the three major etiologic categories of genetic disorders?

   a.

   b.

   c.

5. How does a chromosomal disorder occur?

6. A disruption in the process of _____ , a type of cell division, is the chief cause of trisomies and monosomies.

7. The occurrence of nondisjunction during mitosis results in a numerical change called _____ .

8. Identify the common clinical features of infants born with the following chromosome disorders.

Disorder	Type of Mutation	Common Clinical Features
Trisomy 21		
Trisomy 18		
Trisomy 13		
Turner Syndrome		
Triple X Syndrome		
Klinefelter Syndrome		

9. A chromosomal abnormality might be suspected for an individual who reports an exposure to one of the following environmental agents known to induce chromosomal breaks or other damage.

    a.

    b.

    c.

10. List the four patterns of inheritance and specify a syndrome that occurs as a result of a disorder in that pattern of inheritance.

    a.

    b.

    c.

    d.

11. What is a multifactorial disorder?

12. Identify three ethnic groups for whom carrier screening programs are encouraged.

13. During the assessment portion of a health visit, a woman of childbearing age reports that she has experienced multiple miscarriages. The nurse notes the need for a referral for genetic counseling. What other factors in a woman's personal history or within a family history would indicate a need for genetic counseling?

14. List the five steps in the process of genetic counseling.

15. List skills that are important for a nurse who is involved in genetic counseling, preconception counseling, or prenatal care that includes a focus on screening for anomalies.

Chapter 14

Termination of Pregnancy

STUDY OBJECTIVES

1. Review the history and controversies related to termination of pregnancy.

2. Discuss the responsibilities of the nurse and the employer in health care agencies in which termination procedures are performed.

3. List reasons why women choose to terminate pregnancy.

4. Identify relationships of maternal age, gestational age, and pregnancy status to morbidity from termination procedures.

5. Identify procedures for termination of pregnancy and complications that can occur.

WORKSHEET

1. Complete the following paragraph about the history of termination of pregnancy.

Evidence of instrumentation for induced abortion for pregnancy termination is noted as early as the era of ancient _____ and _____. The first Supreme Court ruling regarding the right of married people to use birth control occurred in _____; this ruling laid the groundwork for the landmark case regarding abortion. The premise that women have a right to privacy in _____ was the basis for overturning a Texas law regarding abortion. This first decision, which occurred in the year _____, gave rise to safe and legal abortion services across the United States and removed restrictions on places where abortions could be performed, allowing the development of clinics dedicated to the care of women seeking abortion services.

Several decisions have taken place with regard to abortion services, including those addressing _____ in 1977 and 1980, _____

in 1979, and _____

in 1981 and 1990. More recent supreme court cases have allowed for certain state restrictions. In _____, a mandatory waiting period and counseling that discourages women from choosing abortion were the result of a ruling that emerged from a case in Pennsylvania. The focus of cases

heard in 1993 and 1994 was _____

_____.

While individuals hold many differing opinions regarding induced abortion for the termination of pregnancy, there are two major viewpoints that drive the call for legal decisions regarding this issue: (1) _____

_____

and (2) _____

_____.

AWOHNN provides a position statement regarding reproductive services that upholds and respects the rights of individual women to choose abortion and designates the rights and responsibilities of the nurse related to abortion and sterilization procedures. The nurse has certain responsibilities, which include _____,

_____, and

_____.

In addition, the nurse has an obligation to inform her employer, at the time of employment, of attitudes and beliefs regarding abortion and sterilization. The employer should be expected to maintain policies for

_____

_____.

2. List reasons why women choose abortion:

   a. _____

   b. _____

   c. _____

   d. _____

3. Certain trends in choices and outcomes are expressed as statements of relationship. Specify the direction of the relationships (positive or negative) in the following statements.

_____ There is a relationship between the age of the woman and the weeks' gestation at which she seeks to obtain an abortion. The younger the woman, the later in gestation she is likely to seek services. The older the woman, the earlier in gestation she is likely to obtain an abortion.

_____ The risk of the abortion procedure increases as the woman's age increases. This is also true for the gestational age of the fetus: risk to the woman increases as gestational age increases.

_____ Multifetal pregnancy reduction (MFPR) is a procedure that has resulted from the increased use of assisted reproductive techniques. MFPR is performed to improve the outcomes of pregnancy based on a known relationship: maternal and fetal morbidity decrease when there are fewer fetuses.

4. Many factors influence the decision regarding the termination procedure to be performed. However, the stage of pregnancy is a primary factor in this decision. Identify the trimester of pregnancy in which each of the following procedures is likely to be done.

Procedure	Trimester(s)
Curettage	
Intra-amniotic Instillation	
Hysterotomy	
Hysterectomy	
RU 486	

5. _____ is the most common complication of termination procedures. List five other potential complications.

a. _____

b. _____

c. _____

d. _____

e. _____

Chapter 15

Fetal Development

STUDY OBJECTIVES

1. Define selected terms regarding fetal development.

2. Identify the sequence of selected events in fetal development.

3. Discuss principles of teratology.

4. Describe mechanisms of teratogenesis.

5. Identify sources for information about drugs and fetal development.

6. Describe fetal surveillance techniques.

WORKSHEET

1. Match the following terms and definitions.

Term		Definition
_____ Gametogenesis	A.	Substance needed to facilitate neonatal breathing
_____ Zona pellucida	B.	The enzymatic process that allows for penetration of the ovum
_____ Surfactant		
_____ Teratogen	C.	The process of transport for large molecules, such as Immune gammaglobulin G.
_____ Pinocytosis	D.	Maturation of sex cells
_____ Syncytium	E.	The outer layer of the trophoblast that secretes the placental hormones of pregnancy
_____ Capacitation	F.	The membranous lining around the egg cell
_____ Facilitated diffusion	G.	An agent that increases the chances of a structural or functional abnormality
_____ Simple diffusion	H.	The process of transfer across the placenta for oxygen, carbon dioxide, water, and most electrolytes
_____ Active transport	I.	The process by which glucose is transferred across the placenta
	J.	The process of transport across the placenta that requires energy

2. Number the following events in fetal development in order of occurrence.

   ____ Blastocyst   ____ Quickening

   ____ Surfactant develops   ____ Fertilization

   ____ Nidation   ____ Capacitation

   ____ Heart begins to beat   ____ Blastomere

   ____ Face appears human   ____ Umbilical cord apparent

3. Discuss these principles of teratology.

   Dose-effect

   Critical moment

   Teratogenic agents produce specific, characteristic malformations.

   Susceptibility is dependent on both the agent and the conceptus.

   Agents that do not harm the mother may still harm the fetus.

4. Based on these principles, how would you instruct a woman during an early prenatal visit regarding teratogens?

5. List the common mechanisms of teratogenesis.

6. Identify two sources of information about the effects of drugs during pregnancy.

7. The developmental period of greatest susceptibility to the effects of teratogens is _____.

8. Complete the following table of fetal surveillance techniques.

Assessment Technique	When Test Is Performed (Weeks' Gestation)	Purpose of Test
Doppler flow studies		
Chorionic villus sampling		
Percutaneous umbilical blood sampling		
Maternal alpha-fetoprotein screening		
Ultrasound		
Amniocentesis		

Chapter 16

Physiologic Changes of Pregnancy

STUDY OBJECTIVES

1. Identify presumptive, probable, and positive signs of pregnancy.

2. From patient data, calculate the expected date of confinement or the advancement of pregnancy using Nagele's and McDonald's rules.

3. Identify physical changes in pregnancy.

4. Describe the reactions involved in pregnancy testing, and discuss the confidence with which results can be utilized.

5. Identify specific physiologic effects of altered hormonal levels in pregnancy.

6. Identify physiologic adaptations in pregnancy that will be detected in routine assessment.

7. Define the supine hypotensive syndrome.

8. List the danger signs that should be reported to a health care provider.

9. Identify clinical and social situations that place the patient at risk of negative perinatal outcomes.

10. Discuss short- and long-term outcomes of care during pregnancy, and describe patient and provider factors that might influence these outcomes.

WORKSHEET

1. Identify the following signs as presumptive, probable, or positive signs of pregnancy.

   _____   Positive pregnancy test.

   _____   Movement of the fetus reported by the mother

   _____   Chadwick's sign

   _____   Breast sensitivity

   _____   Missed menstrual period

   _____   Ballottement of the fetus

   _____   Fetal heart tones

2. In the prenatal clinic, several women attend for confirmation of pregnancy. The physican asks that you calculate the EDC.

   a. What is the EDC?

   b. How is the EDC calculated?

   c. Specify the EDC for the following LMPs.

      February 15, 1997_____

      December 23, 1996_____

      July 4, 1997_____

      November 30, 1996_____

3. Using McDonald's rule, calculate the duration of pregnancy in weeks and lunar months for the following fundal heights.

   10 cm _____

   25 cm _____

   32 cm _____

4. There are multiple physical changes throughout pregnancy. Match the names of the physical signs and assessments in Column A with the appropriate definition in Column B.

Column A	Column B
____ Chadwick's sign	A. The softening of the isthmus of the uterus in the lower uterine segment
____ Goodells' sign	
____ McDonald's sign	B. The upward rebounding of the fetus against the uterus
____ Ballottement	C. Purplish or bluish coloration of the cervix, vagina, and vulva caused by vasocongestion
____ Quickening	
____ Leopold maneuvers	D. A series of maneuvers, accomplished via abdominal palpation, that give information regarding fetal presentation, position, presenting part, attitude, and descent
____ Hegar's sign	

E. The easy flexion of the fundus of the uterus toward the cervix

F. The maternal perception of fetal movement

G. The softening of the cervix and vagina

5. Complete the following paragraph about pregnancy tests by inserting the correct term in the blanks or circling the correct response.

Pregnancy tests detect the presence of _____ in

the urine or blood. This hormone is secreted by the _____

_____, and (is, is not) detectable very soon after concep-

tion. The seven categories of pregnancy tests, namely _____,

_____, _____,

_____, _____,

_____, and _____,

are based on the antigenic property of this hormone, or on the use of

radioiodine.

6. Discuss the terms *false-positive* and *false-negative*.

7. The false-positive and false-negative rates for home pregnancy tests are presented in the text. Do these rates fall within an expected range for laboratory tests? (Hint: You may need to explore the terms *sensitivity* and *specificity of physiologic tests* to discuss these ranges.)

8. Identify the hormone that influences each of the following physiologic changes during pregnancy.

   Anti-insulin effect (or insulin resistance) _____

   Decreased diastolic blood pressure _____

   Relaxation of pelvic joints and ligaments _____

   Increased pigmentation of the skin_____

   Prevention of menstruation _____

   Increased metabolic rate _____

   Augmentation of the intensity of contractions during labor _____

   Softening of the cervix and increased mobility of pubic joints _____

9. Identify the direction of change for each of these physiologic adaptations of pregnancy.

   Heart rate _____

   Cardiac volume _____

   Systolic blood pressure _____

   Diastolic blood pressure _____

   Cardiac output _____

   Rate of respiration_____

   Urine output _____

10. Define the supine hypotensive syndrome, and discuss why this syndrome is a concern during pregnancy.

11. Every pregnant woman should know the signs that should be reported to the health care provider. These 12 danger signs are:

    1. _____   7. _____

    2. _____   8. _____

    3. _____   9. _____

    4. _____   10. _____

    5. _____   11. _____

    6. _____   12. _____

12. From the following patient situations, identify those circumstances that present a risk for the client. Place a checkmark in front of any situation that is a pregnancy risk, and underline the characteristic or status that places the patient at risk.

_____ At her first prenatal visit (at 11 weeks' gestation), Stacy states that she is experiencing urinary frequency.

_____ Roberta calls the hospital. She is frightened because there is a pool of bright red blood on the chair where she was sitting. She denies pain and states that she is due in 6 weeks.

_____ Jennifer is pleased to hear the fetal heart and to be told that her pregnancy is progressing well. Jennifer would like to stop smoking, but has not been able to reduce the number of cigarettes she smokes each day.

_____ Marcia attended "preparing for pregnancy" classes before she conceived, and has taken vitamins with additional folic acid regularly to maintain her health. She exercises regularly, and she plans to continue teaching her 6th grade class throughout her pregnancy.

_____ Monica knows that she is overweight and reports difficulty with her blood pressure. As a single mother of two other children, Monica is already struggling to provide adequate food and housing for her family. Monica's mother used to live with her and "helped with the kids and meals," but her mother left suddenly to stay with a relative who is very ill, and Monica is alone.

13. List short-term and long-term outcomes that can be used to evaluate the effectiveness of care during pregnancy.

Short-term:

Long-term:

14. Discuss how the following factors might affect the outcomes of care during pregnancy.

The competence of the nurse in evaluating the patient's status

The compliance of the patient in attending prenatal assessment visits

The quality of the assessment of the patient's history and health status

The teaching provided regarding the physical changes that occur during pregnancy

Chapter 17

Psychological Responses to Pregnancy

STUDY OBJECTIVES

1. Discuss various theories regarding the developmental tasks of pregnancy.

2. Identify nursing diagnostic statements and assessment techniques that address the woman's response to pregnancy.

3. List factors that influence the degree of acceptance of a pregnancy.

4. Identify behaviors that occur, by trimester, to evaluate the progress of prenatal attachment.

5. Describe the phases of paternal attachment and behaviors specific to each phase.

6. Identify styles of paternal involvement.

7. List activities to facilitate sibling adjustment to the pregnancy.

8. Discuss the significance of the maternal-grandmother relationship.

9. Identify nursing interventions that might facilitate prenatal attachment in high-risk situations.

WORKSHEET

1. Match the following clinical observations (Column I) with the theory or theories that may provide guidance for practice (Column II).

Clinical Observation or Problem

Theory That May Assist the Nurse

1. ___ Nancy, who was recently married, confides that she was not ready for a pregnancy; however, she and her husband are trying to ready themselves and their families for the baby.

2. ___ Helen is eager to learn all the health practices that will fulfill her goal of a healthy newborn.

3. ___ While Jackie was eager to experience pregnancy and have a child, she reports that her partner does not share her excitement. He judges he may never be ready to have children, and has been sullen since learning of the pregnancy.

4. ___ Robin expresses her excitement when the midwife allows Robin to listen to the fetal heart sounds. Robin says, "This is everything I ever wanted; to be a mother is the fulfillment of all my dreams."

A. Pregnancy is a maturational or developmental crisis; it thus represents a critical period in which a normal situation in the life cycle alters one's equilibrium.

B. Deutsch described pregnancy as the fulfillment of the most powerful wish of a woman.

C. According to the Resiliency Model of Family Stress, family adjustment in response to a stressor varies along a continuum from bonadjustment to maladjustment to crisis. Components such as the nature of the pregnancy, the family's resources, and the family's appraisal of the pregnancy influence the outcome.

D. Ensuring safe passage is one of four maternal tasks identified by Rubin.

2. Technologic advances have influenced the information that can be provided to the pregnant woman to verify healthy progress through pregnancy. These advances also provide the nurse with additional opportunities to explore the woman's response to the pregnancy.

Write a nursing diagnostic statement that addresses psychological response to pregnancy for each of these patient interactions and/or observations.

Mary remains very still during the ultrasound exam. In spite of the technician's animated and excited attention to the well fetus at 25 weeks gestation depicted on the scanner, Mary does not react verbally. There is also no change in affect.

Diagnosis_____

_____

Factors you wish to assess further:

Faye is excited as she arrives for her appointment. She thinks she has felt quickening, and is eager to have you confirm her perception. She is beginning to prepare a nursery and to make decisions about infant feeding and care.

Diagnosis_____

_____

Factors you wish to assess further:

Kathy reacts negatively as you weigh her. She is at 34 weeks' gestation, and she has been concerned about her weight throughout her pregnancy. Kathy has not exceeded the expected weight gain at any of her prenatal visits, but often refers to herself in a negative light, certain that she will never be thin again.

Diagnosis_____

_____

Factors you wish to assess further:

3. List five factors the nurse should assess to evaluate the degree of acceptance of a pregnancy.

   a.

   b.

   c.

   d.

   e.

4. List behaviors that can be observed or explored during an assessment to evaluate prenatal attachment in each trimester of pregnancy.

   First trimester

   Second trimester

   Third trimester

5. List the three major phases of paternal attachment and the behaviors that are observable in each of these phases.

Phase	Behaviors

6. Identify the style of paternal involvement indicated by the following observations or interactions.

_____ You ask Linda if she plans to attend childbirth classes. She tells you that her husband does not think they are necessary, but encouraged her to go if she wanted. Her husband, Joe, has not attended any prenatal visits.

_____ Kathy is excited that her partner is helping with the nursery.

_____ Matt is in attendance at each prenatal visit. He asks as many questions as Marta does about her care, her diet, and her progress.

7. From your knowledge of childhood development, suggest some activities for a child of the following ages to prepare for a new sibling. (A childbirth educator may be able to help you with some activities for children of varying ages.)

Age 2 _____

Age 4 _____

Age 6 _____

Age 8 _____

8. Discuss the significance of the maternal-grandmother (the baby's grandmother) relationship to emotional adjustment to pregnancy.

9. Amy experienced repeated miscarriages preceding her current pregnancy. While this pregnancy has advanced further than any of the other pregnancies, Amy verbalizes anxiety about the outcome. She confides that she has been reluctant to prepare for the baby, and wonders what she did in previous pregnancies to cause the pregnancy loss. What measures could the nurse enact to assist in prenatal attachment?

Chapter 18

Sociocultural Aspects of Pregnancy

STUDY OBJECTIVES

1. Identify approaches to assess cultural and religious practices that may influence a woman's behavior during pregnancy and childbearing.

2. Describe ways in which the nurse can support a patient's cultural practices within the health care system.

3. Identify behaviors that indicate that a woman is in the process of maternal role attainment.

4. Define the term *couvade*.

WORKSHEET

1. Assessment of cultural and religious practices that might influence a woman's health behavior during pregnancy is an important aspect of care. List several ways in which a nurse can assess for these customs.

2. Your patient informs you about the customs of her family and culture, and asks how she can assure adherence to specific customs regarding her pregnancy, delivery, and infant child care while she is in the hospital. While these practices are not consistent with the current practices at the hospital, they will not jeopardize the safety of the mother or infant, and they do not conflict with any policies regarding care. What process could you follow to provide the woman and her family with care that is consistent with her customs?

3. For the following observations or interactions, identify the process of maternal role development by placing the correct letter in the column labeled **P** and the behavioral manifestation of that process by placing the correct number in the column labeled **B**.

Process

A. Taking-on
B. Taking-in
C. Letting go

Behavioral Manifestation

1. Mimicry
2. Role play
3. Fantasy
4. Introjection-projection-rejection
5. Identity
6. Grief work

P	B	Observation or Interaction
		During a home visit, Kathy verbalizes that she finally feels capable of providing care for her infant.
		Joanne volunteered to assist in the church nursery, hoping she would "gain some experience."
		Although she is only in her second trimester of pregnancy, Rita has already planned that she and her "little girl" will go to the ballet often, and that her daughter will enjoy dancing.
		As Joanne's pregnancy advances, she talks with women to learn about their experiences "working vs. staying at home." Joanne vacillates with regard to her decision. At varying times, she can envision herself in either role, while at other times, she is convinced that one or the other is best.
		Rita reflects on the freedoms she had as an adult without children.
		As soon as her pregnancy was confirmed, Karen called her friend to go shopping for maternity clothing.

4. Define the term *couvade*.

Chapter 19

Promoting a Healthy Pregnancy

STUDY OBJECTIVES

1. Discuss the significance of health teaching during pregnancy to a woman's long-term health and the health of her family.

2. Distinguish minor discomforts from health problems.

3. Provide rationale and instruction for women experiencing minor discomforts of pregnancy and for women who need assistance with health maintenance.

4. Calculate body mass index and use this data to recommend weight gain throughout pregnancy.

5. Describe the pattern of desired weight gain by trimester.

6. Provide instruction and means of evaluation of effectiveness to patients with questions regarding specific health concerns.

WORKSHEET

1. Why is pregnancy known as a time in the life of a woman when many "teachable moments" occur?

2. For each pair of patient interactions or observations, circle the observation or statement that indicates a minor discomfort, and place an X over the observation or statement that presents a health problem that must be referred to the primary care provider. Provide an explanation to the patient for the occurrence of the discomfort and some advice for relief of the minor discomfort of pregnancy.

"I feel a lot of pressure to urinate. If I don't empty my bladder frequently, I get very uncomfortable."

"I have burning and pressure. It hurts so much when I urinate that I avoid attempts to empty my bladder. My urine is darker than usual, too."

Reason for minor discomfort:

Instructions to patient:

Sally reports nausea and vomiting daily. There is no change in the specific gravity of her urine; her skin and mucus membranes appear well hydrated and pink, and she has gained 2 pounds since her visit 4 weeks ago. Sally's friend suggested that she eat a cracker before getting out of bed, but this has not helped Sally.

Sally reports nausea and vomiting daily. Her urine is concentrated, her skin and mucus membranes are dry, and she has lost weight for the last two prenatal visits. Sally says everything she has tried has not helped to relieve this problem.

Reason for minor discomfort:

Instructions to patient:

Barbara tells you that her legs have been aching, and she has noticed some swelling of her ankles and feet. She denies any area that is particularly painful. When her legs are examined, no areas of redness or warmth are found. The Homan's sign is negative. There is slight dependent edema.

Barbara tells you that her legs have been aching, and she has noticed some swelling of her ankles and feet. She is able to point to an area on her right calf that is particularly painful. The area is red and warm. The Homan's sign on her right leg is positive. She has more edema on the right leg than on the left.

Reason for minor discomfort:

Instructions to patient:

Helen says "You know, one thing that I didn't expect was an increase in drainage." Upon questioning, Helen reports vaginal drainage that is thick and yellow. She also reports an odor and has experienced burning and itching. An examination confirms the thick, yellow drainage. The perineum is red and excoriated.

Reason for minor discomfort:

Instructions to patient:

Jackie, who is near the end of her first trimester, called the office to ask about "fainting episodes that she has been having." She denies any bleeding or pain. She reports that this happens more often when she has been standing a long time or when she changes position; for instance when she stands after sitting for a while.

Reason for minor discomfort:

Instructions to patient:

It is Beth's second pregnancy, and she is now in her third trimester. Beth reports that she is having contractions. She has not kept any record of how often they occur, and she assumes they are false labor. She asks if these are normal.

Reason for minor discomfort:

Instructions to patient:

Helen says "You know, one thing that I didn't expect was an increase in drainage." Upon questioning, Helen reports vaginal drainage to be thin and slightly yellow. She denies perineal discomfort. On examination, the presence of thin vaginal drainage is evident. There is no redness or excoriation on the perineum.

Jackie, who is near the end of her first trimester, called the office to ask about "fainting episodes that she has been having." She denies any bleeding, but reports that all day she has been experiencing pain in her lower abdomen, and it is getting worse. She has not had a problem with fainting until today. She also reports feeling weak and notices that her heart is racing.

It is Beth's second pregnancy, and she is in her third trimester. Beth reports that in the last 2 days, she has been having contractions that have been getting increasingly stronger and more frequent. Today, the contractions are occurring even more frequently. She estimates they occur every 12 minutes. She has also noticed that she is passing some bloody mucus.

4. What is the pattern of weight gain that should be observed?

First trimester _____

Second trimester _____

Third trimester _____

5. Define the following terms:

Pica

Lactose intolerance

6. Body mass index (BMI) is judged to be a better indicator of nutritional status than weight alone. The reason for this statement is demonstrated in this exercise. *The formula for calculating BMI is weight (in kilograms) divided by the height (in meters) squared (weight/height²).* Using the recommendations in Table 19-5 (page 520), suggest the weight gain goal for each of these women.

Sally
Weight 140 lbs. _____ Kg

Height 5'8" _____ meters

BMI _____

Recommended weight gain _____

Debbie
Weight 140 lbs. _____ Kg

Height 5'0" _____ meters

BMI _____

Recommended weight gain _____

Judy
Weight 110 lbs. _____ Kg

Height 5'4" _____ meters

BMI _____

Recommended weight gain _____

Jane
Weight 110 lbs. _____ Kg

Height 5'0" _____ meters

BMI _____

Recommended weight gain _____

Martha
Weight 225 lbs. _____ Kg

Height 5'10" _____ meters

BMI _____

Recommended weight gain _____

Mary
Weight 165 lbs. _____ Kg

Height 5'3" _____ meters

BMI _____

Recommended weight gain _____

7. What is the Kegel muscle?

8. Betty tells you that she has been trying to do Kegel exercises on a regular basis. She wonders how she can assess whether she is doing them correctly and whether they are having their desired effect. What guidance would you give her?

9. Diane indicates that she has been feeling especially tired lately. She relates this feeling to a number of stressful situations at work. Diane asks if you have any suggestions for stress management.

   a. What interventions can you recommend?

   b. What resources can you provide to Diane regarding these interventions?

   c. How can Diane evaluate the effectiveness of these measures?

10. Diane asks what the impact of stress can be on her pregnancy. She says "I realized that I am not making decisions for my health alone, and that many decisions I make are influencing someone else" (she pats her abdomen as she concludes her statement). "I want to understand the consequences if I allow these stresses to continue unmanaged."

11. Based on your understanding of teratology, how would you advise Toni, who reports having a glass of wine and smoking a pack of cigarettes each day? (Review Chapter 9.)

Chapter 20

Perinatal Education

STUDY OBJECTIVES

1. Identify the overall goal of perinatal education.

2. Identify the contributions of various individuals to education for pregnancy and childbearing.

3. List the organizations that influence maternity care services and establish standards for perinatal education.

4. Define and describe preconception counseling and care.

5. Define the cognitive, affective, and psychomotor domains, and plan a teaching strategy for two aspects of perinatal care that employ all three domains.

6. List assumptions held by health care providers and consumer advocates that promote prepared childbirth.

7. Identify the three components of Lamaze prepared childbirth classes.

8. Identify outcomes of prepared childbirth education.

9. Identify the paced breathing strategies utilized in labor, the goal of each strategy, and the reasons for choice of strategy at a given time in labor.

WORKSHEET

1. What is the goal of perinatal education?

2. Each of these individuals contributed to the development of perinatal education. Identify the contribution of each.

   a. Grantley Dick-Read

   b. Velvovsky, Platonov, and Nikoloyev

   c. Lamaze

   d. Marjorie Karmel

   e. Elisabeth Bing

   f. Robert Bradley

3. Name the two organizations that exist to influence maternity care services.

   a.

   b.

4. Preconception care and counseling is a goal of *Healthy People 2000*. How can preconception classes assist in positive perinatal outcomes?

5. Define the following domains of learning.

   a. cognitive

   b. affective

   c. psychomotor

6. Multiple domains are often involved in the learning process. For these two teaching goals, identify the cognitive, affective, and psychomotor content that must be addressed.

   a. *Comfort measures in labor*
      Cognitive

      Affective

      Psychomotor

b. *Breastfeeding*
   Cognitive

   Affective

   Psychomotor

7. Health care providers and consumer advocates who promote prepared childbirth hold several assumptions. One assumption is the belief that birth is a normal, natural, and healthy process. List 5 more assumptions.

   a. _____

   b. _____

   c. _____

   d. _____

   e. _____

8. The three components of Lamaze prepared childbirth classes are:

   _____

   _____

   _____

9. Measurement of outcomes is an important component in managing quality of health care. What outcome measures can be evaluated to assess the effectiveness of prepared childbirth education?

10. Identify the goal of each of these paced breathing strategies, and suggest when the patient may want to utilize each of these techniques.

Paced Breathing Strategy	Goal	Reasons to Employ This Strategy
Slow-Paced Breathing		
Modified-Paced Breathing		
Patterned-Paced Breathing		
Traditional Pushing		
Controlled Exhalation Pushing		

Chapter 21

High-Risk Pregnancy

STUDY OBJECTIVES

1. Define a high-risk pregnancy.

2. Explain the purpose of classifying pregnancies as high- and low-risk.

3. State the two basic causes of spontaneous abortion.

4. Differentiate first trimester losses from second and third trimester losses.

5. Identify high-risk disorders by the common presenting signs and symptoms.

6. Distinguish monozygotic and dizygotic twins.

7. Define and describe a vasovagal reaction.

8. Describe the use of methotrexate in the treatment of ectopic pregnancies.

9. Describe follow-up care after termination of a molar pregnancy.

10. Differentiate preeclampsia from gestational hypertension.

11. Describe the contribution of vasoconstriction to hypertension.

12. Describe changes in clinical data with an occurrence of preeclampsia.

13. Discuss the rationale, risks, and nursing assessments related to the administration of $MgSO_4$ in the treatment of preeclampsia.

14. Describe the pathway of Rh isoimmunization.

15. Define *preterm delivery* and indicate causes and nursing care for patients at risk.

16. Differentiate gestational diabetes and diabetes in pregnancy.

17. Indicate usual and target blood glucose levels and insulin requirements for women with diabetes during pregnancy.

18. Identify the predicted infant size based on the classification of diabetes in pregnancy.

19. Discuss detection of abuse in perinatal settings.

20. Prepare diagnostic statements and assessment criteria for women experiencing high-risk pregnancy.

WORKSHEET

1. Define *high-risk pregnancy*.

2. Risk assessment tools are used to assess level of risk. What is the purpose of classifying pregnancies as high- or low-risk?

3. What are the two basic causes of spontaneous abortion?

   a.

   b.

4. How do first trimester losses differ from those that occur in the second and third trimesters?

5. Describe the use of Laminaria rods in the management of women with abortive losses after 14 weeks' gestation.

6. Describe the symptoms of a vasovagal reaction as might occur during a D & C procedure.

7. The following table includes the common presenting signs and symptoms of high-risk disorders. Identify the signs and symptoms by matching them with the corresponding diagnostic name. In addition, place a 1, 2, or 3 beside the letter to indicate the trimester in which the disorder is most likely to occur.

Signs and Symptoms	Disorder
____ Elevated hCG levels, uterine size greater than expected for gestational age, no fetal heart sounds at the expected time	A. Preeclampsia
____ Elevated blood pressure, protein in the urine, and edema	B. Intrauterine fetal demise
____ Absence of fetal movement, absence of fetal heart tones	C. Ectopic pregnancy
____ No increase in fundal height, fetal heart sounds no longer present, regression of pregnancy symptoms	D. Molar pregnancy
____ Uterus is smaller than expected for gestational age; a unilateral, enlarged adnexal mass is detected. HCG levels increase at a slower rate than expected.	E. Hyperemesis gravidarum
____ Intractable vomiting, dehydration, electrolyte imbalance, and lack of maternal weight gain.	F. Missed abortion

8. Discuss the difference between monozygotic and dizygotic twins.

9. Discuss the use of methotrexate in the management of ectopic pregnancies. In the discussion, include rationale for use, side effects, and necessary follow-up.

   a. Description of drug

   b. Rationale for use in ectopic pregnancy

   c. Side effects

   d. Follow-up care

10. Molar pregnancy is a form of gestational trophoblastic disease (GTD) that results from abnormal proliferation of placental trophoblast. Describe the follow-up that is necessary for women who experience GTD.

11. Preeclampsia is one of several hypertensive disorders of pregnancy.
    a. How is preeclampsia different from gestational hypertension?

    b. How does vasoconstriction contribute to elevated blood pressure?

    c. What are the effects of preeclampsia on these data?
       1. Urine output

       2. Platelet count

       3. Edema

       4. Affect

       5. Reflexes

       6. Vision

12. What is the rationale for the use of magnesium sulfate ($MgSO_4$) in the treatment of preeclampsia?

13. What are the risks of the administration of $MgSO_4$?

14. What assessments should be performed routinely to detect the occurrence of the negative effects of MgSO$_4$ therapy?

15. Describe the pathway of Rh isoimmunization from the entry of Rh positive blood into the circulation of an Rh negative woman to the fetal effects of this sensitization.

16. What standard precautions must be followed before administering Rh$_o$(d) Immune Globulin?

17. Define *preterm delivery.*

18. The causes of preterm delivery can be categorized as:

   a. _____

   b. _____

   c. _____

19. What is the nurse's role in the care of a woman who is at risk for preterm delivery?

20. For the diabetic patient who is pregnant, management of diabetes presents special concerns. For each trimester of pregnancy, complete this table of expected changes in extracellular glucose levels and insulin requirements.

	First Trimester	**Second Trimester**	**Third Trimester**
Blood Glucose Levels (Indicate High or Low)			
Insulin Requirements (Increased or Decreased)			
Target Fasting Glucose			

21. For each of the classifications of diabetes in pregnancy, indicate whether the infant size predicted on the mother's health status will be Large (L) or Small (S) for gestational age.

_____ Class A1   _____ Class B   _____ Class H

_____ Class A2   _____ Class C   _____ Class D

_____ Class F   _____ Class R

22. How does gestational diabetes differ from diabetes in pregnancy?

23. What measures can you take in your interactions with the women you provide care for to increase the likelihood that an occurrence or pattern of abuse will be detected?

24. Use the Parker's Abuse Assessment Screen (page 691) to evaluate the assessment of abuse in the setting where you provide care. Describe similarities and differences in the two assessments.

25. Considering the physical limitations of many high-risk conditions, as well as the known risks to the well-being of the pregnant woman and fetus, write four diagnostic statements that may apply to high-risk pregnancy. List observations and questions that will assist in assessing for these diagnoses.

Diagnostic Statement	Observation or Question

Chapter 22

The Physiology of Childbirth

STUDY OBJECTIVES

1. Identify events in the process of labor as one of the following components: passenger, powers, passage, position, or psyche.

2. Identify events that mark the beginning and end of the stages of labor.

3. Define terms specific to the process and physiology of labor.

4. Identify diameters of the fetal head and pelvis that have significance to labor and birth.

5. Discuss three theories regarding the onset of labor.

WORKSHEET

1. One means of identifying the components of the process of labor is to reference the five P's. In the following chart, identify the component of the process of labor for the term in Column A by placing the correct letter in the space indicated. In Column B, write a brief statement of the significance of the term. The first response is provided as an example.

A. Passenger
B. Powers
C. Passage
D. Position (maternal)
E. Psyche

Column A	Column B
_A_ Sutures and fontanelles	Palpation of the sutures and fontanelles assists in identifying the attitude and presentation of the fetus.
____ Cardinal movements	
____ Effacement and dilatation	
____ Obstetric and diagonal conjugates	
____ The suboccipitobregmatic diameter	
____ Increment, acme, decrement	
____ Birth environment	
____ Recumbent or upright	
____ Lie	
____ Lack of self confidence or lack of knowledge	
____ Attitude	

2. Identify the events that mark the beginning and end of each stage of labor.

   Stage 1

   Stage 2

   Stage 3

   Stage 4

3. Define the following terms.

   Uterotropin

   Parturition

4. Complete the following paragraph.

   The smallest diameter of the fetal head is the _____.
   The measurement of this diameter is _____. The _____ is the
   cavity or plane of least dimension. The anterior portion of this plane is the
   _____, and the posterior por-
   tion is the _____. The _____ conju-
   gate is a direct measurement that can be accomplished on vaginal exam.
   From this conjugate, the _____ conjugate can be esti-
   mated. The usual measurement of this conjugate in all pelvic types except
   the platypelloid is _____.

5. Describe three of the proposed theories regarding the onset of labor.

Chapter 23

Promoting Normal Childbirth

STUDY OBJECTIVES

1. Identify assessments, support, and information that can be provided to women who are questioning their labor status.

2. Identify the process that occurs in various stages of labor.

3. State the usual time intervals of the phases of the first stage of labor, and identify the assessed cervical dilatation that marks the beginning and end of each phase.

4. From a report of a laboring patient, determine the progress of labor and the position, presentation, and descent of the fetus; identify assessments that should be completed; and assign appropriate nursing interventions.

5. Identify behaviors that are indicative of labor progress.

6. Identify the nurse's role in preparing the environment for birth.

7. Identify deviations from expected occurrences in specific stages of labor.

8. Discuss the nurse's role in immediate care of the newborn.

WORKSHEET

1. Susan Jones has arrived for her prenatal visit. She is at 38 weeks' gestation, and this is her first pregnancy. Susan says that this morning she has noticed that she is having contractions. The contractions have not been frequent enough to prompt Susan to time them, but Susan wonders if this could be the beginning of labor.

   a. What questions would you ask Susan to enable you to provide guidance to her?

   b. What assessments do you want to perform to assess the presence of labor?

   c. What do you want to assess regarding Susan's knowledge about labor?

2. What process occurs in the first stage of labor?

3. The first stage of labor is divided into phases. An understanding of these phases can assist the nurse in providing care to the laboring patient. Identify these three phases, the duration for a nulliparous and for a multiparous woman, and the cervical dilatation that marks the beginning and end of each phase.

Phase	Duration	Cervical Dilatation
	Nullipara: Multipara:	
	Nullipara: Multipara:	
	Nullipara: Multipara:	

4. Helen arrives at the hospital, certain that she is in labor. Following an interview with the patient, the nurse does a vaginal examination. The nurse reports the following information: 5 cm of dilatation, 100% effacement, contractions every 3 minutes lasting 45 seconds, palpation of the posterior fontanelle on the right side of the mother's pelvis, fetal heart tones of 136 beats per minute, membranes intact, and fetal station of 0.

   a. What phase of labor is Helen experiencing?

   b. From the information above, what do you know about the descent of the fetus?

c. What do you know about the position and attitude of the fetus?

d. What nursing assessments should be done routinely during this phase?

e. What nursing interventions are appropriate during this phase of labor?

f. What behavior changes would indicate a need for additional assessment of Helen's status in labor?

5. Now Helen has an urge to push. Her cervix is completely effaced and dilated.

a. What stage of labor has Helen entered?

b. What event will mark the end of this stage of labor?

c. What are the primary nursing interventions for this stage of labor?

d. What changes will you expect in uterine contractions and fetal heart rate?

e. In addition to attending the patient, the nurse must prepare the environment in anticipation of the birth. What preparations of the environment must the nurse complete during this stage of labor?

6. The third stage of labor follows the birth of the baby.

   a. What are the signs that this stage is advancing spontaneously?

   b. What assessments of the placenta should be conducted?

   c. What are the expected behaviors of the mother during this stage?

   d. What discomforts or physiologic responses does the woman experience?

7. What assessments are necessary in the fourth stage of labor?

8. Gloria delivered a baby boy 30 minutes ago. The nurse assesses maternal vital signs, and finds a pulse rate of 104 and a blood pressure of 110/60.

   a. What assessments should the nurse conduct based on these findings?

   b. Five minutes later, the pulse rate has increased to 128 and the blood pressure is 78/46. What actions and assessments are now necessary?

9. Describe the components of an Apgar score.

   A

   P

   G

   A

   R

10. Infant Male Jones is assessed at 1 minute following birth. He moves all extremities, is pink in color on his trunk and head, but has some bluish coloration on the soles of his feet, his lower legs, the palms of his hands, and his lower arms. He extends his arms and legs in response to loud noises in the delivery area. He has a pulse rate of 140 and a respiratory rate of 40. What APGAR score should be assigned to Infant Male Jones?

11. Describe the process of identifying the infant. Why must this be done in the delivery area?

Chapter 24

Pain Management During Childbirth

STUDY OBJECTIVES

1. Differentiate the pain experienced in labor from pain experienced with medical and surgical conditions.

2. Discuss the nature, physiology, and neural pathways of pain during childbirth.

3. Name and describe the three phases of the pain experience.

4. Discuss theories to explain causation of pain.

5. Discuss the effectiveness of selected interventions for pain in relation to the gate control theory.

6. Discuss childbirth education as a nonpharmacologic pain management strategy.

7. Identify the effects of systemic and regional interventions on the fetus and the progress of labor.

8. Identify narcotic antagonists and treatments for adverse effects of medications.

9. Identify the use of specific regional anesthesia procedures in labor and the nursing assessments and interventions that must be employed.

WORKSHEET

1. Discuss how the pain experience in labor is different from the pain experienced with other medical or surgical conditions.

2. Discuss the nature of pain, the physiologic changes related to pain, and the nerves and pathways involved in the occurrence of labor pain.

	First Stage	**Second Stage**
Location		
Physiologic changes related to pain		
Major nerves involved		
Pathway		

3. Name and describe the three phases of the pain experience.

    a.

    b.

    c.

4. Match the following theories proposed to explain the concept of pain with the description of the mechanism of pain.

Theory

_____ Endogenous biochemical pain theory

_____ Fear-tension-pain theory

_____ Cognitive control theory

_____ Gate control theory

Description of Occurrence of Pain

A. Specific to pain in labor; fear is implicated as a cause of pain. Fear results in excitation of the sympathetic nervous system and increased uterine tension.

B. The individual invokes mental activities such as dissociation or controlled breathing to decrease the awareness of the incoming pain sensation.

C. Pain impulses are transmitted from nerve receptors through the spinal cord to the brain. This pathway can be inhibited by alternative stimulation that interrupts the pathway.

D. A natural pain suppression system functions at the midbrain, medulla, and the spinal cord. This system is stimulated by pain activity.

5. Explain the effectiveness of the following interventions according to the gate control theory:

   a. Counterpressure

   b. Aromatherapy

6. Childbirth education is described as a nonpharmacologic pain management strategy. Provide a rationale that explains this observation.

7. Pharmacologic interventions for pain management can be systemic or regional. For systemic medications, write a statement that describes general concerns in relation to the following.

   a. The fetus

   b. The progress of labor

8. What narcotic antagonist must be available in the event of newborn respiratory depressions when systemic pharmacologic measures have been utilized?

9. The birth of the infant is often the first hospitalization experienced by the mother. The likelihood of adverse reactions to anesthetic agents, such as those used in regional anesthesia, is not known. What precautions and medications should be taken to identify and treat reactions promptly?

10. In this table, indicate the stage and phase of labor in which each type of
regional anesthesia may be used, and the nursing assessments and interventions related to the initiation of that regional anesthetic.

Type of Regional Anesthesia	Stage (and Phase When Appropriate) of Labor	Nursing Assessments and Interventions
Paracervical block		
Epidural		
Pudendal		
Local		

Chapter 25

High-Risk Childbirth

STUDY OBJECTIVES

1. Discuss maternal-fetal transport.

2. Define the terms *malposition, malpresentation,* and *cephalopelvic dispro-portion.*

3. Describe the findings of vaginal assessment and the observations of the progress of labor that lead to suspicion of malpresentations.

4. Define *placenta previa* and identify symptoms that lead to the diagnosis.

5. List the conditions and lifestyle choices that predispose a woman to abruption.

6. Identify the risk of abruption to the mother and the fetus.

7. Provide a rationale for therapies in the treatment of preterm labor.

8. Discuss the monitoring of a woman who experiences premature rupture of membranes.

9. Identify the emergent treatment of a prolapsed cord.

10. Identify causes and treatment for dysfunction labor patterns.

11. Discuss the diagnosis and medical management of an amniotic fluid embolism.

12. Describe procedures to induction of labor and identify the nurse's role in these procedures.

13. Discuss the nurse's role in psychological support in high-risk situations.

WORKSHEET

1. What is maternal-fetal transport?

2. Define the following terms.

Malposition

Malpresentation

Cephalopelvic disproportion

3. Malpresentations are often first suspected during vaginal examination for assessment of progress of labor. Complete the following table of findings during vaginal examination and observations of progress of labor for these malpresentations.

Malpresentation	Findings on Vaginal Exam	Likely Progress of Labor
Brow presentation		
Face presentation		
Breech presentation		
Transverse lie or shoulder presentation		

4. The diagnosis of placenta previa is confirmed by ultrasound examination. What symptom would lead to the suspicion of **placenta previa**?

5. Define the term placenta abruption.

6. List those conditions or lifestyle choices that may **predispose a woman to** abruption.

7. What is the risk to the mother and to the fetus as a result of abruption?

8. Provide the rationale for the use of each of these therapies in the treatment of preterm labor.

Treatment	Rationale
Administration of magnesium sulfate	
Hydration	
Administration of calcium channel blockers	
Bed rest	
Administration of terbutaline or ritodrine	

9. Why are the results of the following laboratory tests important in monitoring a woman with premature rupture of membranes? What values or results should be reported to the physician?

   a. White blood cell counts

   b. C-reactive proteins

   c. Sedimentation rate

10. Name two strategies that must be accomplished to manage a prolapsed cord until a cesarean delivery can be done.

11. Abnormal labor patterns are best detected by plotting cervical dilatation on the y-axis and time on the x-axis. Normative data for this plot, known as a *partogram,* was developed by _____.

12. Complete this table with information regarding the cause and treatment of hypotonic and hypertonic uterine contractions.

Type of Uterine Dysfunction	Potential Causes	Management of Contractions and Likelihood of Vaginal Delivery
Hypotonic contractions		
Hypertonic contractions		

13. Discuss the diagnosis and medical management of an amniotic fluid embolism.

14. Discuss the following means of induction of labor by completing the chart.

Procedure	Rationale for Use	Nurse's Role in Procedure
Amniotomy		
Prostaglandin E_2		
Administration of oxytocin		

15. For most high-risk conditions in childbirth, a part of the nurse's role is prompt recognition of conditions and enactment of protocols to manage or avoid physiologic crises. In addition, the nurse must provide support and care to the woman and her support network of family and friends. Discuss how each of the following goals regarding support of the woman in crises can be addressed.

    a. Anxiety during physiologic crisis

    b. Grief due to the difference in the actual childbirth experience from the anticipated experience

Chapter 26

Fetal Monitoring

STUDY OBJECTIVES

1. Discuss the response of the fetal heart rate to the conditions of normoxia, hypoxia, and anoxia.

2. State the goal of fetal monitoring.

3. Define baseline and periodic changes.

4. Define patterns of periodic changes.

5. Describe the procedures for internal monitoring and external monitoring.

6. Describe the equipment used in fetal heart rate monitoring.

7. Identify baseline and periodic changes as reassuring or non-reassuring.

WORKSHEET

Fetal monitoring provides an opportunity to assess fetal oxygenation and make clinical judgments about the fetus in relation to the progress and events of labor and childbirth. To best understand the response patterns, responses to changes in oxygenation will first be reviewed.

1. What is the expected range for the fetal heart rate?

2. When the supply of oxygen is first decreased, would you expect the fetal heart rate to increase or decrease? (Consider the response of the human cardiovascular system to brief episodes of decreased oxygen in answering this question.)

3. If the supply of oxygen is restored quickly, and if there are no additional hypoxic episodes, would you expect the baseline (or sustained average) fetal heart rate to increase, decrease, or return to the baseline that preceded the episode of hypoxia?

4. If the supply of oxygen is not restored, would you expect the fetal heart rate to increase, decrease, or remain the same? (Consider the response of the human cardiovascular system to worsening hypoxia in answering this question.)

5. If the supply of oxygen is at a lower level for a sustained period of time, what compensatory changes in fetal heart rate might be evidenced? (Consider the response of the human cardiovascular system to a chronic state of hypoxia in answering this question.)

6. What is the goal of fetal monitoring?

7. There are two major categories of fetal heart rate patterns, baseline: heart rate and periodic changes. How is the baseline determined?

8. Define the following baseline changes.
   a. Fetal tachycardia

   b. Fetal bradycardia

   c. Baseline variability

9. Periodic changes are those that occur in response to changes in oxygenation or in central nervous system changes. Match the following periodic changes with their definitions.

    ____ Acceleration

    ____ Deceleration

    ____ Early deceleration

    ____ Variable deceleration

    ____ Late deceleration

A. A rapid decrease in the fetal heart rate and a rapid return to the baseline that may occur during or between contractions; these decelerations are v-shaped (fast onset, fast recovery)

B. A decrease in the fetal heart rate that begins after the onset of the contraction and ends after the contraction has ended

C. Deviations of the fetal heart rate below the baseline rate that persist for at least 10 to 15 seconds but for less than 2 minutes

D. Deviations that begin at the start of the contraction and end at the same time as the contraction; also described as a mirror image of the contraction

E. Increases in heart rate over the baseline fetal heart rate, usually in response to fetal movement

10. Variability can be identified as short-term variability or long-term variability. Define these terms.

    a. short-term variability

    b. long-term variability

11. Monitoring of the fetal heart rate can be accomplished by external or internal means.

    a. Describe how external monitoring of the fetal heart rate is accomplished.

    b. Describe how internal monitoring of the fetal heart rate is accomplished.

12. Why is the fetal monitor called a two-channel monitor?

13. The fetal heart rate monitor can be used for antepartum fetal monitoring as well as intrapartum monitoring. Describe each of the following antepartum tests.

    a. Nonstress test

    b. Contraction stress test

    c. Biophysical profile

14. Fetal scalp blood sampling is an additional assessment that can be performed to assess the ability of the fetus to compensate for periodic changes that are worrisome. The pH of the blood is assessed for acid-base status. Match the pH values with the interpretation for the fetus.

    ____ 7.20 to 7.25   A. Normal

    ____ 7.19 and below   B. Preacidotic

    ____ 7.25   C. Acidotic

15. Interpretations of fetal heart rate monitoring data in antepartum and intrapartum testing are labeled "reassuring" and "non-reassuring." For the following list of observations, place an "R" when the pattern is one in which no intervention is required, and "NR" for those patterns for which interventions to reduce or relieve hypoxia may be initiated.

    ____ Persistent late decelerations during the active phase of labor

    ____ Present short-term variability

    ____ A reactive nonstress test

    ____ A negative contraction stress test

    ____ A biophysical profile score of 10

    ____ Baseline of 110

    ____ Loss of initial and secondary acceleration

    ____ Variable decelerations during the active phase of labor.

    ____ A non-reactive nonstress test

    ____ Absent short-term variability

Chapter 27

Principles of Family-Centered Maternity Care

STUDY OBJECTIVES

1. State the philosophy of family-centered maternity care.

2. Identify assumptions regarding the family members as a part of a family-centered philosophy.

3. Discuss the role of the nurse in family-centered maternity care.

4. Compare the care in the practice setting where you are with the care that is based on a family-centered philosophy.

5. Generate a plan to address discrepancies and to support similarities identified when comparing practice with a family-centered philosophy of care.

WORKSHEET

1. State the philosophy of family-centered care.

2. Identify assumptions made as part of a family-centered philosophy about the family members and their motivations, participation, and level of involvement in the childbearing process.

3. Identify aspects of the nurse's role that are emphasized in family-centered maternity care.

4. Consider the births that you have witnessed to date. Compare the decision making environment, level of participation and control exerted by the childbearing family, and continuity of care observed in that situation with the empowerment, decision making, participation, and continuity of care espoused in family-centered maternity care.

   a. List the perceived similarities in the philosophy and the reality.

   b. List the perceived differences in the philosophy and the reality.

   c. If differences exist in the philosophy and the observed reality, list some actions that could be taken to increase family-centeredness.

   d. If the philosophy and observed reality are very similar, suggest supportive actions that will sustain the level of involvement offered to families during childbearing.

Chapter 28

Postpartum Adaptation

STUDY OBJECTIVES

1. Describe the process of involution.

2. Discuss the change in lochia during early postpartum adaptation.

3. Provide a rationale for the neuromuscular and sensory alterations experienced in the postpartum period.

4. Distinguish between postpartum blues and postpartal depression.

5. Discuss the physiologic adaptations during the postpartal period and the length of time that the return to the nonpregnant state will take.

WORKSHEET

1. Name and describe the three processes that must occur for involution of the uterus to take place.

   a.

   b.

   c.

2. Specify the term that should be used to characterize each type of lochia described. Indicate the usual time of appearance in the postpartal period.

Appearance of Lochia	Name	Usual Time of Appearance
Dark red to brownish red		
Brownish color, thinner in consistency		
Thick and white or yellow		

3. List some reasons why assessments of neuromuscular and sensory adaptations may be altered in the postpartum period.

4. Discuss the difference between postpartum blues and postpartum depression.

5. Each of the following maternal systems experiences physiologic adaptation during pregnancy and must therefore return to a nonpregnant status. The duration of this change varies with each system. Complete the following chart for changes within each system. The system of concern is indicated in the first column. In the second column, write the time of return to the nonpregnant state and the assessment that would verify this return. In the last column, indicate any intervals in this recovery process that provide an opportunity for assessment.

System	Time of Return to Nonpregnant State and Verifying Assessment	Interval Points of Assessment
Reproductive system		
• Uterine size		
• Breasts		
• Menstruation		
Cardiovascular system		
• Blood volume		
• Pulse rate		
• Cardiac output		

System	Time of Return to Nonpregnant State and Verifying Assessment	Interval Points of Assessment
Hematologic system		
• Hemoglobin and hematocrit		
• White cell count		
• Platelets		
Respiratory system		
• Respiratory rate		
• $PaCO_2$		
Renal system		
• Kidneys		
• Bladder		
Immune system		
Gastrointestinal system		
• Digestion		
• Bowel function		

Chapter 29

Nursing Care of Mothers

STUDY OBJECTIVES

1. State the intent of the Newborns' and Mothers' Health Protection Act of 1996.

2. For specific patient interactions or observations, identify the adaptation from an unexpected occurrence, provide a rationale for the adaptation, and provide instruction for the patient in relation to the change.

3. For selected discomforts that occur in the postpartal period, list interventions for relief and a rationale for each intervention.

WORKSHEET

1. What is the intent of the Newborns' and Mothers' Health Protection Act of 1996?

2. For the following patient interactions or observations, circle the observation or statement that indicates the expected postpartum adaptation, and place an X over the observation or statement that indicates a problem or delay in postpartum adaptation that must be referred to the primary care provider. Provide a rationale for the adaptation and any instructions that should be given to the patient to continue or enhance adaptation.

Jill says she has been to the bathroom to void quite frequently on the first day after delivery. There is no burning associated with voiding. Her temperature is 99° F, pulse 60, and respiration 24. She also notes that the swelling in her ankles is decreasing.

Jill says she has been to the bathroom to void quite frequently on the first day after delivery. She states she has burning and pressure. Her temperature is 101° F, pulse 112, and respiration 28. She feels ill and pays little attention to the infant or to her own general recovery.

Rationale for change:

Instructions to patient:

Michelle recently arrived in her room from the recovery area. She is excited about the baby and her delivery. When first assessing Michelle's uterus, you have difficulty locating the fundus. The fundus becomes firm with massage, and is midline and slightly below the umbilicus. Michelle states she has not voided yet.

Rationale for change:

Instructions to patient:

Barbara tells you that her legs have been aching. She is pleased to note that she can see her ankles and feet, and they don't even look very swollen. She denies any area that is particularly painful. When her legs are examined, no areas of redness or warmth are found. The Homan's sign is negative.

Rationale for change:

Instructions to patient:

Ginger calls from home. She delivered 5 days ago. She is concerned about a change in her vaginal drainage. Yesterday the drainage she noted was light pink, but today it is more red. She said that, in general, she was feeling much better and more energetic today, so she took a long walk and did some housework.

Rationale for change:

Instructions to patient:

You make a routine follow-up call to Mary's house. John, Mary's husband, says that Mary would prefer that you call later. He describes her as weepy and tired. He stayed home today so that she could get some rest, and she is sleeping now. When you question John further, he indicates that Mary has been trying to do too much. He reports that her appetite is fine, and she enjoys holding and caring for the baby.

Rationale for change:

Instructions to patient:

Michelle recently arrived in her room from the recovery area. She is excited about the baby and her delivery. When first assessing Michelle's uterus, you have difficulty locating the fundus. Even though the fundus becomes firm with massage, the fundus is deviated to one side and does not stay firm. Michelle states she has not yet voided.

Barbara tells you that her legs have been aching, and she has noticed some swelling of her ankles and feet. She is able to point to an area on her right calf that is particularly painful. The area is red and warm. The Homan's sign on her right leg is positive.

Ginger calls from home. She delivered 5 days ago. She is concerned about a change in her vaginal drainage. Yesterday the drainage she noted was light pink, but today it is more red. She said that she has not been feeling well and says that she has some lower abdominal tenderness.

You make a routine follow-up call to Mary's house. John, Mary's husband, says that Mary would prefer that you call later. He describes her as weepy and tired. He stayed home today so that she could get some rest, and she is resting now. When you question John further, he indicates that Mary has not shown much interest in the baby. She does not eat, and she has not been sleeping well.

3. Complete this table related to discomforts, measures of relief of those discomforts, and rationale for the effectiveness of these measures.

Discomfort	Measures for Relief Discomfort	Rationale for Intervention
Episiotomy pain		
Hemorrhoids		
Sore nipples • Breastfeeding • Not breastfeeding		
Breast engorgement • Breastfeeding • Not breastfeeding		
Afterpains		

Chapter 30

Newborn Adaptation

STUDY OBJECTIVES

1. Describe the processes of initiation and establishment of respiration, including the internal and external stimuli involved, and the egress of fluid from the alveoli.

2. Identify mechanisms that result in increased or decreased surfactant.

3. Identify the structures and shunts involved in fetal circulation.

4. Discuss the transition from fetal to newborn circulation.

5. Discuss the effect of hypoxia on neonatal circulation.

6. Identify physiologic adaptations in the neonatal period, normal values that should be obtained on assessment of these adaptations, and alterations that require immediate attention.

7. Identify mechanisms of heat loss.

8. Discuss the sensory adaptation of the newborn.

9. Define *habituation.*

WORKSHEET

1. The initiation of respiration is a result of multiple stimuli. Name the external and internal stimuli that induce respiration.

Internal	External

2. The egress of lung fluid is one process that helps establish respiration. Describe the passage of this fluid. Indicate where the fluid leaves the body and the amount that is eliminated at each point of exit.

   a.

   b.

3. What circumstances might alter the prompt removal of this fluid?

4. What is surfactant?

5. For the following situations, place an I on the line indicated for those that *increase* surfactant production and a D on the line for those that *decrease* surfactant production.

   ____ Gestational age > 36 weeks   ____ Thyroid hormone

   ____ Insulin   ____ Corticosteroids

   ____ Estrogen   ____ Perinatal asphyxia

6. Name the three structures involved in fetal circulation and describe the changes that result in the transition to neonatal circulation.

Structure	Change That Occurs with Closure

7. Which of the following shunts has a risk of remaining open if the infant is hypoxic?

8. Identify the following mechanisms of heat loss by matching them with ways in which this mechanism commonly occurs in the newborn.

Mechanism of Heat Loss

____ Conduction

____ Convection

____ Evaporation

____ Radiation

Way in Which Infant Is Exposed to Heat Loss Mechanism

A. Occurs with the exposure of a wet body surface.

B. Heat is transferred to a distant, cooler surface, such as a window or wall.

C. Contact with a mattress, blanket, scale, or warming table that has not been prewarmed.

D. Circulating air in the room, moving air across the infant's skin

9. Each of these systems experiences physiologic adaptation in the first days of life and must make a transition to achieve stability. The duration of this change varies with each system. Complete the following chart for changes within each system. The system of concern is indicated in the first column. In the second column, list the normal values for assessments of these systems. In the third column, list any alterations that require immediate attention.

System	Normal Values for Assessment of the System	Alterations Requiring Immediate Attention
Respiratory system • Pattern		
• Rate		
Cardiovascular system • Blood volume		
• Pulse rate		
Hematologic system • Hemoglobin and hematocrit		
• White cell count		
• Platelets		
Hepatic system		
Renal system • Kidneys		
• Bladder		

Table continues on following page

System	Normal Values for Assessment of the System	Alterations Requiring Immediate Attention
Immune system		
Gastrointestinal system • Digestion • Bowel function		

10. Jane is asking many questions about her baby. She asks when the baby can see, hear, taste, and feel pain. List some ways in which you can demonstrate the status of these senses to the mother. How would you advise her about developing these skills?

11. Jane listens intently to your teaching. You demonstrate the infant's response to sound by using a bell. Jane is concerned that the infant does not respond after the bell has been rung repeatedly. What is this lack of response?

Chapter 31

Neonatal Assessment

STUDY OBJECTIVES

1. Discuss the use of the Apgar score in assessing of the newborn's physiologic status.

2. Describe assessment of the newborn cardiovascular system.

3. Calculate weight loss and determine if loss is within expected limits.

4. Discuss the purpose of girth and circumference measures in the newborn.

5. Identify characteristics of a full-term infant on the Ballard Assessment.

6. Define selected terms related to the assessment of a newborn infant.

WORKSHEET

1. The Apgar score provides a quick assessment of the newborn's need for intervention in the first several minutes after birth. Discuss the meaning of the score at 1 and 5 minutes.

   1 minute:

   5 minutes:

2. Describe the assessment of the cardiovascular system in the newborn.

   a. For what time period should the heart be auscultated?

   b. What pulses should be assessed?

   c. Is blood pressure a usual component of the cardiovascular system? Explain.

3. Infant Female Gray was born 24 hours ago. The birthweight was 7 lb. 4 oz. Today the weight is 6 lb. 15 oz. Is this weight loss within the expected range? Show your calculation.

4. Repeat the calculation for a birthweight of 8 lb. 8 oz. and a 24-hour weight of 7 lb. 12 oz.

5. Discuss the purpose of doing the following measurements.

Measurement	Purpose of Measurement
Abdominal circumference	
Chest circumference	
Head circumference	

6. From the Ballard Assessment, identify those characteristics that are typical of a full-term, mature infant by placing a checkmark on the line beside those characteristics.

    ____ Skin creases on 2/3 of the infant's foot.

    ____ Ear pinna are flat and stay folded.

    ____ The angle elicited in the square window assessment is 0°.

    ____ Lanugo is absent.

    ____ While holding the hips on the exam table, the examiner is able to touch the ear with the heel.

    ____ Male genitalia are pendulous and have deep rugae. In the female, the labia majora completely covers the labia minora.

7. The higher the score assigned on the Ballard Assessment, the more mature the newborn. Is this observation a positive or negative relationship?

8. Define the following terms.

Acrocyanosis

Jaundice

Cephalhematoma

Thrush

Syndactyly

Meconium

Chapter 32

Nursing Care of Newborns

STUDY OBJECTIVES

1. For specific observations of newborn behavior, response, or adaptation, describe interventions to be performed, give a rationale for the intervention, and indicate teaching that the parent or parents should receive regarding the occurrence.

2. Differentiate physiologic and pathologic jaundice.

3. Identify assessments related to infant feeding.

4. List instructions regarding care of the infant.

5. Explore values and prepare unbiased, non-judgmental responses to care situations in which the expression of opinion or bias is likely.

WORKSHEET

1. During a feeding, Infant Female Hughes begins gagging. Attempts to clear the airway without suction are not effective.

   a. Describe the procedure for using the bulb syringe to clear the airway.

   b. Joan Hughes wants to learn to clear the airway. What procedure will you teach her?

   c. In clearing the airway, should the mouth or nose be cleared first?

2. Joan asks about Sudden Infant Death Syndrome. She has been reading that it is better to place the baby on her back for sleep, but Joan's older sister has been telling Joan that babies are at less risk on their "bellies."

    a. What advice can you provide to Joan?

    b. What could you advise regarding a response that Joan can give her sister?

3. Baby Male Campbell has had problems with temperature regulation. Karen is eager to unwrap her baby, Sean, so that she can "check out his fingers and toes."

    a. How will you instruct Karen about heat loss? What mechanism of loss will occur if Sean remains unwrapped and exposed to air?

    b. Karen said the doctor told her that additional glucose monitoring is necessary today. Karen asks if the temperature and glucose are related. Provide an explanation for Karen.

    c. Karen asks if this problem will continue, and starts to cry. "I don't even have a thermometer at home, and I won't know what to do!" What will you tell Karen about the likelihood of this problem continuing?

    d. What support and instruction can you provide to Karen regarding monitoring the temperature?

4. Describe the relationship between liver function and the vitamin K injection administered after birth.

5. What is the purpose of the eye treatment administered after birth?

6. Certain occurrences in the newborn's early extrauterine life may increase the likelihood of pathologic jaundice. Name some of the predictors of pathologic jaundice.

7. The nurse practitioner asks you to obtain a bilirubin measurement. Describe how bilirubin can be assessed.

8. You report the bilirubin level obtained from an invasive measure of bilirubin. The nurse practitioner asks you to initiate measures to avoid a further increase and to obtain an additional measurement in 12 hours. What measures should you initiate?

9. The bilirubin is increased at the next assessment. The nurse practitioner judges that it would be best to implement phototherapy. What safety measures and protocols will you employ to assure a safe and effective treatment?

10. Jessica Richards is attempting to feed her infant. You elect to remain with her to observe her technique, to observe the infant's response, and to provide support and teaching as needed. Jessica makes several attempts to initiate feeding. The infant is very sleepy and disinterested. Because Jessica is attempting to breastfeed and there has not been an attempt at feeding in more than 3 hours, both you and Jessica want to have a successful feeding episode.

    a. What can you assess for signs of readiness for feeding?

    b. What rationale can be provided for the frequency of feedings? (Address the significance to both the mother and the infant.)

11. Providing factual information to families about the care of the infant is an important part of the nurse's role in providing care to the newborn. Complete the following chart with important details about infant care that you will want to include in your instructions.

Topic	Advice and Instruction
Elimination	
Feeding	
Cord care	
Bathing	
Safety	
Clothing	

12. Decisions regarding methods of feeding and procedures such as circumcision are rooted in family, cultural, and religious values. While the nurse may have strong feelings or opinions about what would be best for the nurse and for the nurse's family, these feelings and opinions should not be expressed as advice to the mother, who is vulnerable in decision making. For the following situations, prepare a response that is non-judgmental and unbiased.

a. Abbie says she is undecided about a circumcision for her new son, but her husband feels strongly this should be done. She asks what you would advise. She has been reading that it is an unnecessary procedure.

b. Nathaniel feels strongly that breastfeeding is the best method of feeding for an infant, and wants Marty to breastfeed their new daughter. Nathaniel and Marty have had a number of discussions about this, and they continue to disagree. Marty has agreed to try breastfeeding, but does so reluctantly. She is having difficulty at a feeding at which you are assisting. She says, "I never wanted to do this anyway—don't you think I should quit?"

Chapter 33

Breastfeeding

STUDY OBJECTIVES

1. Explain historical and current trends in breastfeeding.

2. Discuss the importance of breastfeeding.

3. Explain the lactation process.

4. Identify barriers to breastfeeding.

5. Discuss nursing interventions that promote successful breastfeeding.

6. Develop a plan of care for common breastfeeding problems.

7. Discuss research questions that focus on approaches to improve the rate of breastfeeding.

WORKSHEET

1. The *Healthy People 2000* health status objective for breastfeeding is to increase the number of mothers who breastfeed their babies in the early

   postpartum period to _____ percent, and to increase the number of mothers who breastfeed their babies until they are 5 to 6 months to

   _____ percent.

2. Name the four populations identified by *Healthy People 2000* that should receive special efforts to increase the rate of breastfeeding.
   1.

   2.

   3.

   4.

3. The World Health Organization provides a list of 10 steps for promoting successful breastfeeding to agencies that provide maternity and newborn care services.
   a. These 10 guidelines form the basis for the _____ initiative.

   b. List the 10 steps.
      1.

      2.

      3.

      4.

      5.

      6.

      7.

      8.

      9.

      10.

4. Complete the following table with the appropriate breastfeeding rates.

Date	In Hospital	At 6 Months
1930s/1940s		NA
1970s		NA
1984		
1993		

   NA = Not Available

5. A reporter for the community newspaper asks you to summarize (briefly, because of word limitation for the article) the trends in breastfeeding. What will you say?

6. You are at a party and meet a woman who is pregnant. During your conversation, she tells you that she is undecided about breastfeeding. She asks you why it is better to breastfeed. What will you tell her?

7. Compare the composition of colostrum, mature breast milk, and infant formula.

Factor	Colostrum	Breast Milk	Infant Formula
Bioavailability			
Fat type and content			
Lactose			
Iron			
Immunoglobulins			
Hormones			
Enzymes			

8. Explain the effect of colostrum on the breastfed infant's level of circulating bilirubin.

9. A friend tells you that she has decided not to breastfeed because she has to return to work when the baby is six weeks old. What will you tell her?

10. Label the figure of the physiologic process of breast milk production and explain each step in the cycle.

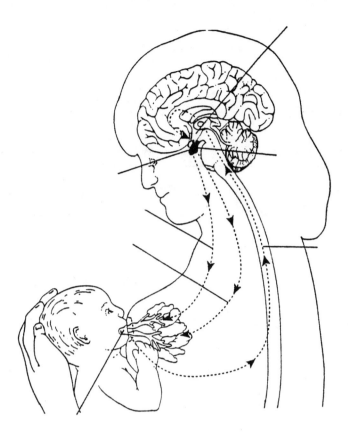

11. List the four general barriers to breastfeeding and give several examples of each barrier.

12. Describe the 13 interventions that form the nucleus of breastfeeding care.

13. You are caring for a new mother who had a cesarean birth, and she is putting the baby to the breast for the first time. Describe two positions for breastfeeding that would be the most comfortable for her. List the steps you should use to assist the baby to latch on to the breast.

14. Sally gave birth to a 5-pound, 3-ounce healthy infant of 36 weeks' gestation. She has difficulty waking her baby up to breastfeed. After a few sucks at the breast, the baby falls back to sleep. Her baby sleeps most of the time and rarely cries when he is hungry. What is a likely cause of Sally's breastfeeding problems? Develop a plan of care for Sally and her infant to promote successful breastfeeding.

15. Susan complains of severe nipple pain while breastfeeding. What should your initial assessment include? List appropriate interventions for this situation.

16. Compare engorgement, plugged milk ducts, and mastitis by completing the following chart.

	Engorgement	Plugged Milk Ducts	Mastitis
Cause			
Symptoms			
Treatment			

17. Alan, born at 30 weeks' gestation, will be ready to go home from NICU in about one week. His mother pumped her breasts and provided breast milk for his feeding until he was able to nurse at the breast. Alan has been nursing at the breast for almost two weeks now. What breastfeeding information does Alan's mother need prior to discharge?

18. You have been asked to plan an exhibit to promote breastfeeding at a community health fair. Design the exhibit and explain what you will do. Who will you select to help you? What resources will you include? Describe how your exhibit will promote breastfeeding.

Chapter 34

Parenting the Healthy Infant

STUDY OBJECTIVES

1. Discuss historical and contemporary social factors that have influenced parenting behaviors.

2. Describe the concepts of bonding and attachment.

3. Identify factors that influence the development of parent-infant attachment.

4. Discuss the concepts of parental role attainment.

5. Review strategies and tools that can be used by nurses to assess early parent relationships.

6. Identify adaptive and maladaptive mothering and fathering behaviors.

7. Identify strategies and tools that nurses can use to assess infant behaviors and infant temperament.

8. Review nursing interventions that can promote positive parent-infant relationships.

9. Identify special needs of adoptive, adolescent, and single parents, and parents of twins.

10. Identify research questions related to the promoting of positive parent-infant attachment.

WORKSHEET

1. Match the concept in Column A with the appropriate statement in Column B.

    Column A

    A. Bonding

    B. Attachment

    C. Reciprocity

    D. Acquaintance process

    Column B

    ____ Develops gradually during the child's first year of life

    ____ Reciprocal process

    ____ Primarily unidirectional (parent to infant)

    ____ Rhythmic cycles of attention and nonattention

    ____ Occurs during the first hours or days after birth

    ____ Interaction between parents and infants during the early days and weeks after birth

2. Complete the following chart by listing factors affecting parent-infant attachment.

Variables	Specific Factors
Parental variables	
Situational variables	
Infant variables	

3. Define *maternal role attainment.*

4. Explain the four stages in the process of parental role acquisition.

5. Name six ways in which the mother influences mother-infant attachment. Which of these maternal factors has the greatest influence on mother-infant attachment?

6. Name six ways in which the infant influences mother-infant interaction. Which of these infant factors exerts the greatest influence on mother-infant interaction?

7. Identify each maternal behavior as adaptive (A) or maladaptive (M).

_____ Talks to baby

_____ Smiles at baby all the time without change in affect

_____ Uses animal characteristics to describe baby in a negative way: "He looks like a monkey."

_____ States relief that baby is of the desired sex

_____ Asks questions about caring for infant

_____ Supports infant's trunk and head while holding the infant

_____ Minimal amount of talking to infant while he/she is sucking

_____ Refuses to leave baby with someone else

_____ Arranges for someone else to take baby in for medical checkup

_____ Makes specific observations about baby

8. Describe the progression of maternal touch as the mother becomes acquainted with her infant.

9. Name six categories of interventions for promoting healthy parenting. Give specific examples of what you would do for each category.

Chapter 35

Alterations in the Health Status of Postpartum Mothers

STUDY OBJECTIVES

1. Discuss the role of the nurse in caring for postpartum patients experiencing a medical complication or cesarean delivery.

2. Identify the most common alterations (complications) in the postpartum period, including their definition, incidence, etiology, and clinical manifestations.

3. List factors that predispose a woman to develop complications such as hemorrhage, infection, thrombophlebitis, and psychological disorders in the postpartum period.

4. Discuss medical management of patients with the most frequently occurring postpartum complications and the role of the nurse in the implementation of this management.

5. Identify common infections during the postpartum period.

6. Explain the importance of being familiar with risk factors for postpartum complications.

7. Suggest possible nursing diagnoses and the corresponding goals, nursing interventions, and outcome evaluation measures for postpartum hemorrhage, infection, thrombophlebitis, and psychological disorders.

WORKSHEET

1. Answer the following questions about postpartum hemorrhage.

   a. What amount of blood loss constitutes postpartum hemorrhage?

    b. What are the three criteria for severe postpartum hemorrhage?

        1.

        2.

        3.

    c. What are the two classifications of postpartum hemorrhage? What feature distinguishes between the two?

    d. What is the most common cause of postpartum hemorrhage?

    e. During what time period does a woman have the greatest threat of postpartum hemorrhage?

    f. What should you do *first* if you suspect that a woman is bleeding too much following delivery?

2. List the predisposing risk factors for uterine atony.

3. You are caring for a postpartum woman who is having excessive bleeding. Describe two methods of estimating blood loss. Which one is more accurate?

4. What is a hematoma? What are the symptoms of the different types of hematomas?

5. Describe the three types of abnormal placental attachment.

6. What are the symptoms of retained placental fragments? Describe the management of retained placental fragments.

7. Describe two ways in which postpartum bleeding differs from uterine atony and lacerations.

8. Name five things you should assess when caring for a woman with thrombosis.

   1.

   2.

   3.

   4.

   5.

9. List the symptoms of pulmonary embolism. Why do the symptoms vary among individuals?

10. What is the criterion for the diagnosis of puerperal infection?

11. List the three factors that are responsible for the majority of puerperal infections.

    1.

    2.

    3.

12. Describe the signs and symptoms of postpartum infection.

13. Complete the following chart to identify the factors that increase a woman's risk of postpartum infection in the antepartum and intrapartum periods.

Time Period	Factors
Antepartum	
Intrapartum	

14. What do parametritis and peritonitis have in common? What are the differences between the two conditions?

15. Compare the signs and symptoms and treatment for breast fullness, breast engorgement, and mastitis.

16. Complete the following chart on postpartum affective disorders.

Disorder	Signs/Symptoms	Treatment
Postpartum Blues Onset and Duration		
Postpartum Depression Onset and Duration		
Postpartum Psychosis Onset and Duration		

17. Mark the following statements true (T) or false (F).

_____ Approximately 50 to 80 percent of all postpartum women experience postpartum blues.

_____ Postpartum infection can occur without an elevated temperature.

_____ The most common cause of early postpartum hemorrhage is retained placental fragments.

_____ Approximately 10 percent of all postpartum women develop thrombophlebitis.

_____ Postpartum infection is the leading cause of maternal morbidity and mortality.

_____ If a woman has a firmly contracted uterus but continues to bleed heavily, lacerations of the cervix, vagina, or uterus should be suspected.

_____ The majority of women with postpartum hemorrhage have predisposing risk factors.

_____ Changes in pulse rate and blood pressure are early indicators of postpartum hemorrhage.

_____ During the immediate postpartum period, bladder distention is a common cause of uterine atony.

_____ The condition in which the uterus has a slower return than normal to its prepregnancy status is termed _involution_.

_____ When measuring bleeding using the gram scale, one gram equals 5 mL of blood.

18. Match the symptoms or lab results in Column A with the appropriate condition in Column B.

Column A	Column B
A. Increased fibrin degradation products	_____ Uterine inversion
B. Blood loss often underestimated by as much as 50 percent	_____ Disseminated intravascular coagulation
C. Profuse bleeding with abdominal pain	_____ Mastitis
D. Tenderness and pain in lower extremity	_____ Puerperal infection
E. White blood cell count of 13,000 on second postpartum day	_____ Postpartum hemorrhage
F. Unilateral, localized breast tenderness	_____ Thrombophlebitis

Chapter 36

Alterations in Health Status of Newborns

STUDY OBJECTIVES

1. Discuss high-risk conditions for the newborn including their etiology, risk factors, signs and symptoms, interventions, and implications.

2. Discuss the classifications of the newborn according to gestational age and weight.

3. Describe the difference between major and minor anomalies.

4. Describe appropriate nursing interventions for congenital anomalies recognized in the newborn period.

5. Discuss the etiology, incidence, and potential outcomes of some commonly recognized congenital anomalies.

6. Discuss the nursing process as it relates to the high-risk infant and family.

WORKSHEET

1. Define preterm infant, post-term infant, and term infant.

    a. Preterm infant

    b. Post-term infant

    c. Term infant

2. Complete the following table on the SGA, LGA, and AGA infants.

	Definition	Cause	Physical Characteristics	Nursing Care
SGA Infant				
LGA Infant				
AGA Infant				

3. What size nasogastric tube should you use for gavage feeding an infant?

4. Explain how you would check the nasogastric tube for correct placement.

5. Describe the three levels of perinatal care within a regionalized perinatal care system.

6. Where are the Level III and Level II perinatal care centers in your state?

7. What two things are absolutely essential for effective care when an infant has to be transported to a tertiary care center?

8. Complete the following table on the complications of respiratory distress in the preterm infant. List one specific nursing diagnosis for each complication.

Complication/Nursing Diagnosis	Cause	Symptoms	Nursing Care
Pulmonary Hemorrhage			
Pulmonary Interstitial Emphysema			
Pneumothorax			
Bronchopulmonary Dysplasia			

Complication/Nursing Diagnosis	Cause	Symptoms	Nursing Care
Intraventricular Hemorrhage			
Enterocolitis			
Necrotizing Entercolitis			
Patent Ductus			
Sepsis			

9. State the four *initial* steps in the *correct order* for resuscitation of the newborn.

    1.

    2.

    3.

    4.

10. Describe three problem areas that require special consideration in caring for the preterm infant.

11. What is the "safe" level of bilirubin in the preterm infant as compared to the full-term infant?

12. Develop a plan of care for the infant of a diabetic mother.

13. What is kangaroo care and how is it used in the NICU?

14. Explain the differences between an omphalocele and gastroschisis.

15. What is the one most important symptom of esophageal atresia in the newborn infant?

16. Which infants are more likely to have anorectal agenesis?

17. What factor determines the severity of pulmonary compromise in the infant who has a diaphragmatic hernia?

18. What two characteristics are hallmarks of Potter syndrome?

19. What are the differences among anencephaly, myelomeningocele, and hydrocephalus? What do they have in common?

20. Complete the following chart on chromosome disorders in the newborn.

Condition and Cause	Neonatal Characteristics	Expected Outcomes
Trisomy 13		
Trisomy 18		
Trisomy 21		

21. State the two categories of cardiac disorders in the newborn and describe the difference between the two conditions.

22. List 11 types of heart lesions in the newborn and complete the following table.

Heart Lesion/Type/ Pathophysiology	Clinical Findings	Treatment

Heart Lesion/Type/ Pathophysiology	Clinical Findings	Treatment

22. Explain the different grades of heart murmurs.

23. You are caring for an infant who is being worked up to determine if he has a heart defect. In morning report, you are told that the infant's urine output had decreased slightly during the last eight hours. Also, he did not eat well, becoming very tired and unable to finish the bottle feeding. When you are assessing the infant, you note that his skin color is pale and his extremities are cool. What clinical significance do these symptoms have? What should your further assessment include?

Chapter 37

Parenting the High-Risk Neonate

STUDY OBJECTIVES

1. Identify historical trends related to the care of physiologically compromised high-risk infants and their families.

2. Identify common parental reactions to a high-risk pregnancy.

3. List the four tasks that mothers must accomplish to resolve the crisis of the birth of a physiologically compromised infant.

4. Describe the four major categories of stressors that parents encounter at the birth of a physiologically compromised infant.

5. Examine the effects of the birth of a high-risk infant on parent-infant attachment.

6. Discuss the effects of the birth of a high-risk infant on the parents' relationship with one another.

7. Describe common reactions of siblings and extended family members to the birth of a high-risk infant.

8. Assess the level of attachment between parents and their high-risk infant.

9. List potential nursing diagnoses related to high-risk parent-infant attachment.

10. Describe nursing interventions to help parents cope with the birth of a high-risk infant.

11. Develop a plan of care to promote parent-infant attachment and optimum parenting behaviors.

12. Identify questions for future research related to parenting high-risk infants.

WORKSHEET

1. Define the term *high-risk infant.*

2. Mark the following statements true (T) or false (F).

   _____ Any condition that threatens the health or well-being of the mother, father, or neonate can adversely influence the development of parent-infant attachment.

   _____ All parents' reactions to a high-risk pregnancy and birth are similar.

   _____ Prolonged separation of parents and their high-risk infants during the newborn period is a major source of family stress.

   _____ High-risk infants have fewer care-soliciting and social behaviors than full-term, healthy infants.

   _____ Preterm infants usually have difficulty coordinating sucking and swallowing until 32 to 34 weeks.

   _____ The rate of child abuse is the same for preterm and full-term infants.

   _____ Family members usually progress through the stages of grief at about the same rate.

   _____ Grandparents' reactions to a preterm birth are similar to the parents' reactions.

   _____ Siblings' reactions to the birth of a high-risk infant vary with the particular family situation.

3. a. Complete the following sentences.

   A parent's increased ability to care for the high-risk infant reflects

   _____, while the parent's increased satisfaction

   with the infant reflects that _____ has occurred.

   b. How will these observations affect your plan of care for the infant and the family?

4. Why should you encourage each parent to spend some time alone with their infant?

5. Describe the three stages of behavioral development in the preterm infant. At approximately what gestational age does each stage occur? What are the infant's developmental responses during each stage?

6. Name eight behaviors that indicate sensory overload or distress in the preterm infant.

7. Develop a plan of care to promote parent-infant interaction for the preterm infant and the parents. What factors should you consider when developing this plan of care?

8. Explain three ways in which a nurse can help prepare parents for their first visit to their high-risk infant in the NICU.

9. What are the key components of successful intervention programs for parents of preterm infants?

10. Develop a discharge plan and a plan for follow-up for the preterm infant.

Chapter 38

Perinatal Loss and Grief

STUDY OBJECTIVES

1. Identify ways in which perinatal mourning may differ from mourning for other kinds of loss.

2. Differentiate anticipatory, normal, and pathologic grieving.

3. Identify phases of mourning as they relate to perinatal loss.

4. Describe how individual and family characteristics impact perinatal mourning.

5. Identify specific nursing interventions to assist families with perinatal loss.

6. Describe interventions to meet the needs of women and families from special populations.

7. Cite reasons for identifying feelings of loss on the part of caregivers, along with strategies to meet these needs.

8. Identify questions for future research about perinatal loss, grief, and mourning.

WORKSHEET

1. Identify the following statements as true (T) or false (F).

   _____ Individuals may experience feelings of loss and the need to grieve at any time during the childbearing year.

   _____ All grieving mothers who are hospitalized should be transferred off the maternity unit to another area of the hospital.

   _____ The creation of a supportive environment includes some way of identifying the mother (and her room) as an individual that has experienced a loss.

   _____ Preschoolers may feel responsible for their sibling's death.

   _____ A subsequent pregnancy will contribute to the resolution of grief.

   _____ Providing opportunities for parents to care for their dying infant and to hold their infant after death is helpful to most parents.

2. Explain how each factor listed below affects the individual's response to perinatal loss.

Factor	Effect
a. Individual Characteristics	
b. Family Characteristics	
c. Circumstances Surrounding Loss	
d. Interventions to Assist Grieving Individual(s)	

3. Define the three types of perinatal grief, the approximate time frame of each, and characteristic symptoms.

   a. Anticipatory

   b. Normal

   c. Pathologic

4. Match the phase of mourning in Column A with the appropriate statement in Column B.

   Column A

   _____ Yearning/Searching/Anxiety

   _____ Disorganization

   _____ Shock/Disbelief

   _____ Reorganization

   Column B

   A. The initial response to loss; characteristics include apathy, physical detachment, and inappropriate behavior.

   B. Commonly most intense from second week to fourth or fifth month after loss; characteristics include blaming, anger, fear, and physical symptoms.

   C. Intense period of mourning 4 to 6 months after the loss. Characteristics include difficulty in accomplishing normal tasks, despair, and preoccupation with the lost infant.

   D. Restoration of the capacity to interact with others and plan for the future.

5. Name three strategies for helping parents who experience perinatal loss that nurses can use to achieve each of the desired goals listed below.

   a. Validating the loss

   b. Making the loss real

   c. Teaching parents about grief

   d. Helping the grieving woman who is being seen in a physician's office

   e. Providing effective follow-up for perinatal loss

6. Describe four reasons why using a comprehensive checklist for perinatal loss can improve nursing care that is provided for women and their families.

Chapter 39

Adolescent Pregnancy and Parenthood

STUDY OBJECTIVES

1. Examine the problem of adolescent pregnancy and parenthood, including incidence, cultural influences and differences, and factors associated with teen sexual activity.

2. Describe the consequences of adolescent pregnancy and parenthood, including health risks for the mother and infant, psychosocial consequences, and the impact on society.

3. Discuss the different types of adolescent pregnancy prevention programs.

4. Examine issues related to adolescent pregnancy and their implications for health policy and health care programs.

5. Discuss the advantages and disadvantages of the choices available to the pregnant teen, including how each choice can be discussed with the teen using a decision-making model.

6. Plan appropriate management for the pregnant teen and adolescent mother in both agency and community settings.

7. Identify risk management strategies when providing care for the adolescent family.

8. Develop research questions related to adolescent pregnancy and parenthood that need to be addressed.

WORKSHEET

1. Answer the following questions.
   a. How many teens become pregnant in the United States each year?

   b. What percent of the adolescent pregnancies are unintended?

   c. What percent of female teens experience a pregnancy before completing high school?

   d. What percent of female teens will give birth to a child while still a teen?

   e. What percent of female teens who get pregnant will have an elective abortion? A spontaneous abortion?

   f. What percent of teenage mothers will become pregnant again within two years after a first pregnancy?

2. Identify the following statements as true (T) or false (F).

   ____ Adolescent pregnancy is a relatively new phenomenon.

   ____ The rates of sexual activity and the age of initiation of sexual activity in the United States are similar to those of other Western developed countries.

   ____ U.S. teens have significantly higher rates of adolescent pregnancy, abortion, and childbearing than their counterparts in almost every other industrialized nation.

   ____ Hispanic teens are more likely to give birth as adolescents than white teens.

   ____ History indicates that reducing adolescent sexual activity and pregnancy is possible.

   ____ The impact of adolescent pregnancy on family relationships is similar for all ethnic groups.

3. What are the factors that influence teens' initiation of sexual intercourse?

   a. Biologic factors

   b. Social factors

   c. Environmental factors

4. Describe specific consequences of adolescent pregnancy and parenthood in the areas below.

   a. Maternal factors

   b. Neonatal factors

   c. Psychosocial consequences

5. Match the type of adolescent sexuality education program in Column A with the appropriate statement in Column B.

Column A	**Column B**
A. Traditional sexuality education	____ The major criticism of this approach is the introduction of the concepts of non-sexual intercourse and homosexuality.
B. Abstinence-only sexuality education	____ The curricula for these types of programs were primarily developed with federal grant money.
C. Abstinence-based/postpone sexuality education	____ Emphasizes reproductive anatomy and physiology and sexually transmitted diseases
D. Comprehensive sexuality education	____ Stresses the acquisition of decision-making and refusal skills

6. List the steps in pregnancy decision-making using a problem-solving approach.

7. Mary, 16 years old, is 8 weeks pregnant as a result of rape. After counseling and careful consideration of her options, she has decided to terminate the pregnancy. Using the Decision Tree (Figure 39-5) on p. 1468, develop a plan of care for Mary.

8. Leeza, a single 17-year-old, "is pregnant" (according to a home pregnancy test she did) with her second child. She has not had a menstrual period since the birth of her first child, a girl, who is 5 months old. She "will definitely keep" the baby and hopes that it is a boy. Using the Decision Tree (Figure 39-5) on p. 1468, develop a plan of care for Leeza.

Chapter 40

Perinatal Infections

STUDY OBJECTIVES

1. Identify the major organisms causing perinatal infections.

2. Describe the modes of transmission of perinatal infections.

3. Describe the risks to the mother of the most commonly occurring perinatal infections.

4. Describe the risks to the fetus/neonate of the most commonly occurring perinatal infections.

5. Describe the nursing actions and responsibilities in the identification and treatment of perinatal infections.

6. Identify the factors that influence preventive measures and treatment regimes for the most commonly occurring perinatal infections.

7. List those infections which are preventable through either active or passive immunization.

8. Describe nursing actions and responsibilities in the prevention of perinatal infections.

9. Develop a teaching plan emphasizing prevention of perinatal infections through active and passive immunization.

10. Identify areas for further research within the realm of perinatal infections.

Complete the following tables for bacterial infections, viral diseases, parasitic diseases, and other perinatal infections.

BACTERIAL INFECTIONS			
Infection	**Mode of Transmission**	**Risks to Mother**	**Risks to Fetus/Neonate**
Chlamydial Infection			
Gonorrhea			
Group B Streptococcus Infection			
Listeriosis			
Lyme Disease			
Syphilis			
Tuberculosis			
Infection	**Signs/Symptoms**	**Prevention**	**Nursing Considerations**
Chlamydial Infection			
Gonorrhea			
Group B Streptococcus Infection			
Listeriosis			
Lyme Disease			

Infection	Signs/Symptoms	Prevention	Nursing Considerations
Syphilis			
Tuberculosis			

		VIRAL DISEASES	

Disease	Mode of Transmission	Risks to Mother	Risks to Fetus/Neonate
Cytomegalovirus			
Hepatitis A			
Hepatitis B			
Hepatitis C			
Herpes Simplex Types 1 and 2			
HIV/Maternal			
HIV/Neonatal			
Human Papillomavirus			
Influenza			
Measles			

Table continues on following page

VIRAL DISEASES			
Disease	**Mode of Transmission**	**Risks to Mother**	**Risks to Fetus/Neonate**
Mumps			
Parvovirus			
Rubella			
Varicella Zoster/ Herpes Zoster			
Disease	**Signs/Symptoms**	**Prevention**	**Nursing Considerations**
Cytomegalovirus			
Hepatitis A			
Hepatitis B			
Hepatitis C			
Herpes Simplex Types 1 and 2			
HIV/Maternal			
HIV/Neonatal			
Human Papillomavirus			

Disease	Signs/Symptoms	Prevention	Nursing Considerations
Influenza			
Measles			
Mumps			
Parvovirus			
Rubella			
Varicella Zoster/ Herpes Zoster			

PARASITIC DISEASES

Disease	Mode of Transmission	Risks to Mother	Risks to Fetus/Neonate
Trichomoniasis			
Toxoplasmosis			

Disease	Signs/Symptoms	Prevention	Nursing Considerations
Trichomoniasis			
Toxoplasmosis			

Table continues on following page

OTHER PERINATAL INFECTIONS			
Infection	**Mode of Transmission**	**Risks to Mother**	**Risks to Fetus/Neonate**
Candidiasis (Yeast Infection)			
Bacterial Vaginosis (Gardnerella Vaginosis)			
Urinary Tract Infection			
Scabies/Lice			
Infection	**Signs/Symptoms**	**Prevention**	**Nursing Considerations**
Candidiasis (Yeast Infection)			
Bacterial Vaginosis (Gardnerella Vaginosis)			
Urinary Tract Infection			
Scabies/Lice			